POSITIVE LIFE SKILLS FOR TEENS

No More Stinky Socks And Smelly Armpits, How To Deal With
A Rollercoaster Of Emotions, Learn Social Skills & Get Good
With Money

REBECCA COLLINS

AUTHOR PROFILE

Rebecca Collins is the mother of two teenagers, a boy and a girl. She is also a highly respected personal development coach. Being the only girl in a family of four brothers, she quickly learned to be tough if she wanted to keep up with the boys.

This go-get-it attitude drove her to set up her own company at the age of 25. After completing a degree in business management, she went on to invest in female start-ups and organized online workshops aimed at enabling women to realize their full potential in both their professional and personal lives.

After several years of coaching, geared towards raising self-esteem and self-confidence in both teens and adults, she decided to put her work into print. Rebecca is also an influential voice in the female empowerment niche. She currently resides in Oxford, England.

Receive Rebecca's Newsletter, FREE "Reclaim Your Power" https:// rebeccacollins.co.uk Please ask your parents or guardian before signing up. All newsletters are aimed at helping people to increase their confidence and self-esteem, you can unsubscribe any time by clicking the link at the bottom of each email.

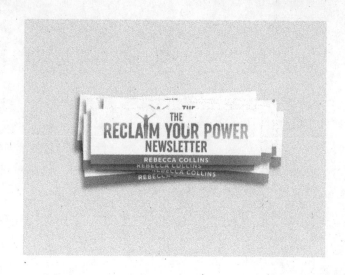

CONTENTS

INTRODUCTION

If you are between 12 and 19, you've probably reached that stage in your life where you think your parents are kinda weird.

One minute, they are telling you to "grow up" and the next, they remind you of how "you aren't old enough" to do this or that. It's a pretty confusing world and here you are, stuck in a kind of limbo: not yet a fully grown adult but certainly NOT a kid.

It can be so annoying and frustrating at the same time. Sure, there's a lot you don't know about life, but that doesn't make you an idiot. There are plenty of things you are capable of doing by yourself and you don't need your parents for everything! Anyway, you probably hate being told you are too young, too immature, or not responsible enough.

So, here's the thing: your parents aren't going to cut you any slack if you don't show them you've earned it. Relying on them for mundane stuff like clean clothes, food on the table, lifts to school, and so on, is great, but it also tells them that you aren't ready to take ownership of the things that concern you. The best way to overcome this is to prove to them that you ARE responsible, that you CAN do a lot by yourself, and that you ARE ready to grow up.

Think of it like a win-win situation: you begin learning basic life skills and your parents will start treating you like a grown-up. Apart from that, which is a bonus in itself, you also get to stand on your own two feet and skill-up on life's essentials like how to deal with money, cook your favorite pizza, organize your free time better, and even learn how to defrost the fridge!

That's what this book is about: teaching you how to do the simple things in life that will stand you in good stead for the future. As well as that, you will learn how to take control of your life now and avoid the constant nagging about your room being a mess, your homework not being done, and hearing over and over again that money doesn't grow on trees.

Seriously? Don't you just want to live a hassle-free life so you can concentrate on chilling out more with friends, be able to buy the things you like with your own money, know that you are at the top of your game with school work, and not have to waste three hours searching your cluttered bedroom for your new earbuds?

You may feel that you have a lot to learn and that school isn't teaching you anything useful. Let's face it: how much use are logarithms really going to be in your future career? The reality is that most schools are designed to give you a general academic education that may or may not be useful in the future. They definitely aren't there to teach you how to invest money or change a tire. These are the kind of things you need to learn from someone else and most likely, your parents don't have the time or energy to do that.

As a working parent who has raised two kids, I know what it's like to come home after a long day at work and have to cook, sort out the washing, organize drop-offs or pick-ups, and have little time to myself. It's frustrating to find a sink full of dirty dishes (and an empty dishwasher just standing there!), smelly socks littering the bathroom, and kids asking for more money to buy PC games or the latest iPhone.

Sometimes, when my kids were younger, I used to feel like screaming, and would often go on a half-hour rant about how they should help more, how I'm not a human cash machine, and how they should "Grow up!"

Parents, I must admit that this is NOT the right way to go about things. Instead of complaining that my kids didn't do anything to help themselves, I began to realize that I hadn't taught them the skills I accused them of not having in the first place. I had to take some responsibility for that and began to implement a different approach, which worked out best for everyone in the long run.

Now, they are both fully functioning responsible human beings who can handle money, survive the day without starving, and definitely know how to defrost the fridge. How did I manage that? You'll find the answers to that in this book.

To young adults reading this book, there are many life skills that you can pick up at an early age and I know you are a quick learner.

- Even a twelve-year-old can understand the benefits of saving money, and teens can easily grasp the fundamentals of starting their own business or securing a good job. A lot of them are already doing it!
- Learning how to look after yourself and take care of your own personal items such as clothes isn't rocket science - anyone can master the art of using a washing machine - honestly.
- Being organized just needs a little planning and once it becomes a habit, everything gets a lot easier. Time management is one of those essentials in life and helps avoid a lot of last-minute dramas. Once you've nailed that, there's no more rushing around at the last minute trying to find school books or being late for football practice for the umpteenth time.
- Learning how to shop for groceries on a budget and still be able to cook a healthy meal is a superpower that you can also acquire with a little guidance and know-how. It can bring you a great sense of satisfaction and also makes you a very resourceful adult. And just appreciating the value of money itself takes you to genius skill level.

It's not only the practical things in life that you need to deal with though. From your early teens, your body is undergoing some epic changes and that's often hard to deal with. The emotional rollercoaster that comes with the shift from young person to adulthood can often make you feel totally miserable. All of a sudden, you have a face full of acne, hate the way you look, can't stand your parents poking into your personal life, and you really just want to fit in.

Adolescence is tough but there are ways to navigate it so that you don't get dragged down by those intensely negative thoughts and emotions.

- Change is a part of life and instead of fearing that you are mutating into some kind of reptilian, you can learn here about getting through the ups and downs in a positive way.
- And if you feel like you have no friends, you will also find lots of tips on how to make new ones and ways to prevent internet trolls from making your life a misery.

You are never too young to start learning basic skills like making and saving money, organizing your time (and bedroom), healthy eating, personal hygiene, and even car maintenance. You'll find all you need here to navigate the weird world of feelings too, with great advice on how to feel good about yourself and adopt a positive body image. It makes no difference if you are a girl, boy, haven't made your mind up yet about your sexual orientation, or whether you are thirteen, fifteen, or seventeen. There are plenty of life skills you can pick up now that will serve you well in the future.

If you are a parent or carer, reading this book will give you some nifty insights into how to avoid conflict with your kids and enable them to become confident, resourceful adults. You can't force them to grow up overnight but you can be there to support them as they learn to stand on their own two feet. You will have the chance to rethink strategies that haven't been working so far and discover new ways to guide them through that rocky transition from childhood to adulthood without the usual tears and tantrums.

But this book is really for teenagers and if you are one, think of it as a user manual on how to deal with the nitty-gritty things in life and give yourself a head start for your future.

Are you ready to power up and take on the world?

Let's go, starting with the one thing that makes it go around - MONEY!

❧ I ❧

GET SMART WITH MONEY -
THE BANK OF MUM AND DAD
IS EXPIRING

Money really does make the world go around, but it's usually the adults who do all of the earning and spending. That also gives them financial control, meaning that you have to ask them every time you want a new pair of sneakers or go to Starbucks with your mates.

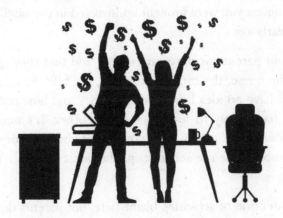

That can be a pain in the neck, especially if they can't afford to meet your demands and, no doubt, you know the lecture off by heart about the importance of money, blah blah blah.

Even if your family are pretty well off, you likely don't have access to money at will, or you could be on a relatively low weekly or monthly allowance. Your pocket money may not be enough to keep you in the latest trendy clothes, or you might have to do chores (which you hate) to earn it. It totally sucks, right?

There's a lot you can do to get around this, but the main thing you have to understand is the value of money. It really isn't an endless stream of dollar bills or pound notes that the ATM machine generously spews out.

It has to be earned, usually by hard work, and it can vanish as easily as it appears. It's not magic - one minute you have it and, if you're not careful, the next minute you can find yourself totally broke.

I don't want to give you a headache but the money issue needs to be sorted out here and now so you can make the most of it later on in life. I want to first ask you a very simple question and see if you know the answer off the top of your head:

How much money does your family earn each month and what are your total household outgoings?

Any ideas? Thought so... it's probably something you've never had to think about unless you were brought up involved in the family finances from a very early age.

You know your parents work to earn money and that they spend it on things like the house, the car, the groceries, the bills, you... right? But you probably have no idea how hard they work and how much money goes in one hand, only to leave out of the other. It's never been a concern of yours so far and all you know is that you need, or want, that new jacket, money for the school trip, the latest tablet.... The list is truly endless.

There's no intention of attaching blame here, but parents don't usually involve their kids in the ins and outs of the family finances. It's kind of seen as an 'adult' thing and most sixteen-year-olds know very little about saving or investing. It could be that you have grown up in a household where money is always tight, so you've never had the chance to experience any kind of real financial management.

It might also be the case that, although your family are wealthy, you've never been interested enough to ask your parents what they do with their money, if they invest, or what goes into financial budgeting.

You don't need to have finished Harvard Business School to know that money opens doors for opportunities you wouldn't otherwise have, aside from putting a meal on the table. And you can start to develop a better relationship with money no matter what age you are, although the younger, the better.

Money equals freedom!

Put it this way: wouldn't you like to start making your own money instead of having to constantly ask your parents for it? It's not just about being able to go to the mall and splash out on a pair of designer sneakers or throwing it away on fast food.

Earning your own money is a game-changer because it makes you appreciate what's needed to get it, and it teaches you to be more careful about how you spend it. That's a very healthy habit to start practicing as soon as possible, and one that will stand you in good stead when you eventually enter the world of adulthood.

But before you reach that stage, just imagine the feeling of having financial freedom...being able to buy what you want without stressing out mom and dad. Even better: how about being able to contribute to the household expenses?

There is no better way of getting your parent's respect than that, and they will definitely appreciate the gesture. It's really liberating to earn your own money, and there are plenty of ways to do it.

My parents didn't have a lot of money while I was growing up so I can't say I was able to keep up with the latest fashion trends, which was a bummer. All of my friends were buying nice clothes (well, I mean their parents bought them...) but I didn't have that option and often felt like the odd one out. Wearing hand-me-downs is a great way to recycle clothes, but I had older brothers, so that was not cool - I didn't feel all that girly in boy's second-hand sweat pants.

When I was fourteen, I found a Saturday morning job in a local bakery. It was kind of fun learning how to make pies (including the secret recipes) but it was more than that: I was on a mission. With the money I earned each week, which really wasn't a lot, I had set myself a goal of buying a new pair of jeans...girl's jeans.

It took me about 6 weeks to collect enough money and I still remember even today that exhilarating feeling of making my first, very own purchase with MY hard-earned cash! Needless to say, it made me feel like I was the same as my other friends and it did wonders for my self-confidence.

At that age, it sucks when you don't feel like you fit in, and nobody wants to be laughed at for their lack of fashion sense or for anything else. It's the same for boys, who also want to feel part of the gang, whether that's through having the latest haircut or a snazzy pair of basketball boots.

I'm not saying that material things are everything, but fitting in really is essential during your teenage years. A lot of kids feel left out, lonely, and socially ostracized, which can have a devastating effect on their physical and mental well-being.

Clothes and gadgets don't build character, buy happiness, or help us to make real friends, but being a part of a group is important when you are 15 or 16. Having some spending power can help you to do that, even if it's to go to the cinema with your mates at the weekend instead of missing out because you can't afford the ticket.

Easy come, easy go

Assuming that you get some sort of pocket money,

- How much do you think you have been given in the last twelve months?
- Did you keep it or spend it?

- What about money you were given from other family members for your birthday, Christmas, or for passing exams?
- How much did you get in total?
- And, more importantly, WHAT DID YOU SPEND IT ON?

You have probably been used to getting pocket money from a young age and like to spend it on eating out at your local fast food restaurant with friends or buying clothes, gadgets, makeup, and personal items, depending on your needs.

Most teens tend to spend money on the same things no matter where they live and wanting to have fun is normal. But at some point, it's good to start thinking about what else you can do with your pocket money and how you can become even more financially smart.

You might have access to your pocket money or allowance through some type of digital banking in an account that has been set up for you by your parents. In the cashless society that we live in, using a bank card to pay for stuff is easy to do, because it doesn't feel like you are really spending any money at all.

You just swipe and go, and that's it! In many ways, it's harder to keep track of what you are spending like this because you never actually *see* the money in your hand.

Making online purchases is also a part of life nowadays and there's a lot of temptation to sign up for things like music streaming services, buy online video games, or fill up your cart with a new outfit at the click of a button.

It's a cool way to shop and everyone does it, but understanding where the money is coming from and keeping tabs on how much you are actually spending is a must.

If you don't appreciate the value of money, it will be a lot harder to hang on to it when you start working or go to college. Now is the time to develop a healthier relationship with money, instead of seeing it as here today, gone tomorrow.

Money is money, no matter how you spend it, but are you using it wisely? It's fine to treat yourself every now and again, but what about other ways to spend your money, or even earn more of it yourself?

How to earn your own money

One of the easiest ways to earn extra money is to help your parents with chores. If you already do that, then you can also expand your entrepreneurial skills with other money-making schemes. Whenever you are offering to do something outside the home for others or online, make sure to get your parents' permission, and always let them know where you are and what you are up to - safety first and foremost!

• Household chores

Getting paid to help around the house might sound like a slow burn but it's a great way to start understanding how real life works: you do a task and get rewarded for it. And no doubt, your folks will be over the moon to see you wanting to lend a hand.

Don't think of it so much as a chore, which is such a negative word these days, but as a chance to fulfill your own needs and desires.

If you normally avoid helping out, remember that it really isn't a big deal and tasks usually take much less time than you imagine. Instead of moaning about them, think of your savings account getting fatter - does that work for you?

Your parents will probably be only too happy to give you even more to do if you offer and show a willingness to learn. Plus, it will get you out of your bedroom for a while to see what's going on in the real world!

• Being a good neighbor

A lot of your neighbors might not have anyone to help them out with things like tidying up the garden or mowing the lawn, especially elderly folk, and that's a great opportunity for you to make extra money. Just pay them a visit and ask what you can do to help.

Tell them you are trying to save up some money and could do with the extra work. You'll probably be warmly received and, as it's in your neighborhood, you don't have to go far or lose time traveling anywhere. It makes good sense, right?

- **Making four-legged friends**

Did you know that people get paid to walk dogs? You don't need any qualifications for that - just a love of animals - and you can make extra pocket money by walking more than one at the same time. Ask around and you could find people in your area who would really appreciate your help and be prepared to pay you a small fee for the service.

You could also offer to pet sit when someone goes on holiday, as long as you feel confident enough to look after their animal. If someone asks you to take care of their baby python though, you may want to rethink that!

- **Elbow grease**

Most people hate taking their car to the car wash because it can be expensive, time-consuming, and such a hassle. That's where you can step in and all you need is a bucket of soapy water, a sponge, and a leather.

Start by cleaning your parent's car, if they have one, and then offer to do neighbors' cars too on a regular basis. With a bit of old-fashioned elbow grease, you can earn a nice little regular income, and even offering to mow their lawn too can be the start of a good money-making project.

- **Watching baby**

If you are responsible enough to take care of a toddler or young child, then you should give babysitting a try. It's a great way to earn extra pocket money and many teenagers rely on a weekend babysitting job to top up their allowance.

In most cases, it involves very little effort and can even be a lot of fun. If you have younger siblings, you already know what's involved and will find it super easy to do.

- **Doing odd jobs**

There's always something to be done around the house so why not offer to lend a hand if you want extra cash? You could discover that you actually enjoy painting walls or fixing broken fences and the more experience you get, the better you will become. It might even be a chance for you to think about a career in carpentry, plumbing, or home decor.

- **Part-time work**

You'll be surprised at how many local businesses are looking for help a few hours or days a week or want seasonal workers. As long as you are at the legal working age and your parents agree, you can start earning good money.

The next time you go to your local stores, pop in and ask if they need any extra help and watch out for job posts on shop windows. As well as gaining experience, you are taking your first step into working life and can reap the rewards!

- **Becoming an eBay wizard**

One person's junk is someone else's treasure and you can sell almost anything on eBay. You can start by sorting through your old PS games, Pokemon cards, or Barbies - anything that you don't use anymore - and put them up for sale on eBay. Someone, somewhere, may be willing to pay a few dollars for them and you can even offer to sell your friends' stuff on their behalf and keep a small commission for yourself.

- **Make it and sell it**

If you like making jewelry or are good at handicrafts, you can easily sell your creations online. Big platforms like Instagram and Etsy let you set up shop for free and buyers can order from you directly.

You may need the help of your parents to do this and with their go-ahead, you can find customers looking for your handmade products. Whether it's hair scrunchies, beaded bracelets, artwork, or homemade cookies, there's plenty of demand for it. Many successful entrepreneurs started out in this way, so why not you?

How to save successfully

If you manage to earn a little money, the next thing to do is learn the value of saving it. Yes, you may feel the urge to go out and spend it all at your local amusement park or blow it on an expensive new laptop, but that's not the best kind of habit to adopt.

I know it's difficult to think about saving when you want to buy that new jacket or camera and the money you have earned is just sitting there. It's normal to want to treat yourself or see the reward for your hard work and you can do that, but blowing all of it in one go just takes you back to square one.

Instead of going on a spending spree, be smart and think about what you need, as opposed to what you want. Do you really need that 500-dollar camera? (£370) Is that 200-dollar jacket a priority? (£150)

If you don't feel that you have learned how to manage money from your parents or the adults in your life, that's OK. You've probably played Monopoly or Minecraft, right?

With games like that, you will have gained some idea about the power of money and know that if you spend it all, it's game over. Here are some tips to help you save and develop that healthy habit of spending wisely:

- **Set a target**

Think about what you would really like to buy and make a realistic savings plan. You can write it down in a notebook or make a spreadsheet, keeping track of how much you have saved, and how much more money you need to reach your goal. It's a great way to stay in control of what you spend and to see your savings get bigger and bigger.

Say you want to buy a new PC screen in six months and it's 500 dollars. How much money do you have now... 30, 50, 150? How much money do you think you can expect to get next month...another 50, 70? Keep a record and see it adding up.

If you don't think you are going to reach your target, talk to mom and dad, as well as older relatives. Tell them you are trying to save and would appreciate their help. By showing them that you are being responsible and trying, you might find that they are willing to meet you halfway or at least contribute something to help you achieve your goals. If you are looking for even more ways to make money, Pinterest has a lot of saving challenges and craft ideas that you can use.

- **Watch what you spend**

You may only spend a dollar here or a dollar there, but very soon you can find that your savings account is empty because it all adds up in the end. It's a great idea to keep a record of what you buy as this helps you to see where your money is going and what you can do to stop that hole in your savings from getting bigger and bigger.

Divide your money into categories such as incomings and outgoings. Then, note exactly what you have spent and next to it, a small review on how useful/necessary it was. You will soon discover that you are spending far too much on snacks, junk food, or useless gadgets that you don't really need.

Even paying for that cinema ticket to see the new Avengers or Spiderman movie can be a waste of money if it's not your thing and by keeping a log, you will soon learn which purchases were a good idea and which weren't. This will stop you from making the same mistakes in the future.

You can download an app on your smartphone to help you keep track of your money, such as BusyKid, Tip Yourself, Mint, and FamZoo.*

There's even an app that lets you plan, save, and budget for your prom night called Plan'it Prom, which can take the stress out of that all-important event!

Some apps may need parental consent, depending on how old you are, so speak to them and find one that you are both happy using.

(*Some apps may be affiliated with certain banks so you need to talk to your parents before setting one up.)

There are also apps like Monzo that lock your money into saving pots, meaning that you can't get access to it until a date set by you. This is a great idea if you can't resist the temptation to break into your savings and it stops you from wasting money on a whim. It may sound like torture but trust me, it's worth it.

- **Go shopping with parents**

You might think this is totally uncool, and I hear you. Who wants to be dragged around the supermarket with mom or dad? What if you are seen by one of your friends? Will you ever live it down? But guess what: mom and dad are usually experts on shopping wisely and you can learn a thing or two about budgeting just by pushing that supermarket trolley around with them.

Most families try to stick to a weekly or monthly budget, so take notice of what they buy - and more importantly - what they don't buy.

Any shopping cart should be filled with produce that is fresh, healthy, and can provide substantial meals, and OK, with one or two snacks to keep you happy (more about the art of grocery shopping to come in Chapter 4 so stay tuned).

The same goes for clothes shopping - notice how your parents shop around, check the labels for price and materials. They are making smart decisions based on value for money + quality - something you should always bear in mind when spending your own money.

Get into investing

This may sound like the big league but plenty of kids and teens have started investing and the earlier you begin, the easier it becomes. There's no secret to investing money and you don't need to be a millionaire or work on Wall Street. For things like formal trading, you do have to be over 18 and will need your parents to handle things until you come of age.

Investing your pocket money or earned income can be as simple as opening a savings account at your local bank. This is what most folk used to do before the world was digitized and youngsters became tech-savvy.

You can start investing now to help out with your college fees, for when you are ready to buy a home of your own or even for retirement (I know this sounds like a million light-years away at the moment, but it isn't). The longer you have to save, the more money you will have at the end of it so time really is on your side, whether you are 12 or 18.

Today, there is plenty of info on the internet to help you learn about investing money and as long as you have some guidance and do your homework, there's no reason why you can't make an extra income. If you are feeling super ambitious, you can even become an entrepreneur like many young adults, making a few bucks by doing one thing then using that money to fund your next venture, and so on.

Remember that there's a difference between saving and investing: people usually save up to acquire something in the future, while they invest to create more money from the money they already have. From your first piggy bank to actually buying shares or trading in bitcoin, there's a lot to learn, so find out as much as you can before you do anything with your money. Just make sure it's legal first!

Read blogs, watch Youtube videos, nag your parents or adults in the know, talk to your friends, and find out as much as you can. If you are able, get some help from a financial professional or visit your local bank and wise up about what investing really means. Learn about trading, the stock market, and starting a business if it interests you and before you do anything, try your hand at gamification apps like How

The Market Works and Build Your Stax, which use fake cash to introduce you to the world of investments.

Cashing in on insurance

Many parents and grandparents set up some kind of insurance policy for their kids or grandkids to provide them with coverage for the child's entire life.

You may have one of your own and, as long as the premiums are paid, it can be a nice thing to have for when you get older. It's often possible at 18 or 21 to take ownership of the policy yourself and you can continue to pay into the policy or cancel it altogether and get a cash payment.

Although this sounds like a great way to get your hands on a whole lot of money, remember that the longer you leave the policy running, the more money it will mean for you in the future. Do you really need to splash out now, or can you do without it and look forward to a nice big pile of cash later on in life? Think carefully about it and make sure to ask for advice from the person who set up the insurance for you in the first place - they will help you to make the right choice.

Playing it safe

You belong to the generation that has grown up with technology and think of yourself as pretty plugged into the digital world. You were probably playing with apps on your tablet or smartphone before you had learned to talk and I'm sure you understand the importance of being careful when online.

Despite that, it's possible that no one has ever really told you about the things you should be looking out for to protect your personal information and money in the virtual world. I want to mention a few need-to-know basics and remind you of what you should be careful of.

- **Social media**

Love it or hate it, you probably use some kind of social media platform to connect with friends and peers. You might use it to chat, exchange photos or videos, follow your favorite celeb, and meet new people. That's all fine, but what about if someone asks for your personal info or banking details? There are a lot of scammers on social media who pretend to be one thing but are really only interested in tricking you into giving them something. You should always be on high alert for that and never share any personal information with someone you don't know or trust.

Your folks may nag you about this all the time and it can be so annoying - you're not stupid, right? The truth is that the more comfortable you are with social media, the easier it is to get complacent and think everyone is your friend, or that you know what you are doing. Beware, because scammers are always one step ahead of you and are experts at fraud and deception.

- **Something smells fishy**

Watch out for those emails asking for your personal information or asking you to click on their bogus website. Make sure you only click on attachments or links if you know where they are from and get anti-virus software on your device. Never give any personal details over the phone either or reply to texts requesting information related to your bank, which are both very common scams these days.

Be careful when shopping online, make sure you buy through an official website because when you give your card details or make a payment through a service like PayPal, you could end up losing all of your savings if the scammers have their way. Scammers are expert at creating copy-cat websites and sending scammy phishing emails to fool people.

Avoiding free public WiFi is also a good idea unless it's an emergency because it can easily be hacked by criminals wanting to steal data such as your passwords and email address.

Talking about money is one of the best ways to learn how to manage it. Your parents may have great money skills or be totally useless. Whatever the case, it's good to learn from them about their mistakes, how their decisions have made an impact on their lives, and what money worries they have.

This will give you a real insight into just how important it is to handle money well and to secure your future. Listen, learn, and spend wisely!

Top tips

- *Earning your own money brings financial freedom, independence, and less parental nagging.*
- *You need to know where money comes from, and how easily it disappears.*
- *Online shopping is the same as using cash - it's all money.*
- *There are plenty of ways to make extra money if you really want to.*
- *Saving money is just as important as making money.*
- *Learning to invest will bring you more money in the future.*
- *Protect yourself from scammers, swindlers, and fraudsters at all times.*

CLEAN UP YOUR ROOM,
CLEAN UP YOUR LIFE

Teens of the world, I know that most of you have messy rooms and hate it when your parents nag you about it all the time.

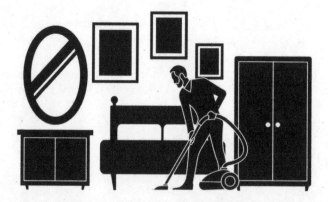

You just can't see their problem: what's it to them if your clothes are lying all over the place, you haven't made the bed for weeks, and you have a collection of mugs growing some kind of green stuff in them?

You don't even notice the moldy smell of wet towels or care if your school books are chucked under the bed, so why should they?

If I was your parent, I'd leave you to it. Yes, it's your space and entirely up to you to keep your bedroom in any state you like. I wouldn't be hassling you 24/7, banging on your door, or nagging you about the mess in your bedroom because I know it doesn't make any difference to you. In fact, it just gets on your nerves. After all, it's YOUR bedroom!

Your room is your safe haven, your little bit of privacy, away from the outside world where people keep telling you what to do all the time. I completely get it. Where else can you break the rules, do what you want, and suffer no consequences if not in your own bedroom? It's your gaming zone, your chat room, your 'friends only' space, and when you close that door on your parents, you are free!

So, just continue to leave your worn clothes piled up in a heap, let those plates with stale food under your bed fester, and don't even think about dusting or cleaning. I know the smell doesn't bother you and you never notice that it looks like a rubbish tip so make it as messy as you want to and don't worry about it. No problem.

Your parents might think I've gone stark raving mad and that I'm totally irresponsible for suggesting such a thing. The truth is, this isn't some kind of reverse psychology or a total lack of concern about the state of your bedroom. It's just a different approach, but I'm sure you'll get it. Read on and you'll see what I mean.

As a teenager, you've got a lot to deal with. Schoolwork, exams, soccer practice, cheerleading routines, all make demands of you. It's too much pressure sometimes, especially when you are trying to come to terms with things like dating, hair growth, spots, dental braces, and greasy hair.

After a long day at school or at weekends, all you want to do is watch YouTube videos, chat on your smartphone, play some online games, catch up with your favorite series on Netflix, or sleep. The last thing on your mind is worrying about those dirty boxer shorts littering the floor or the collection of chocolate wrappers all over your desk.

You will be used to having fights with your mom and dad about this by now and know what they are going to say every time they come into your room. The conversation usually goes something like this:

Mom: When are you going to clear up this mess?

You: It's my room and I'll do what I want.

Mom: Wrong! It's our home and you have to live according to our rules!

You: Why does it bother you what my room is like?

Mom: Because I want it to be clean. It's unhealthy and embarrassing.

You: It's not embarrassing to me. What's all the fuss about!

Dad: If you don't get it cleaned by tonight, there's no more internet for you.

You: Yeah, right. That's not going to happen.

Dad: You'll do what we tell you, or else...

You: Why can't you give me a break? I'm so over this.

Door slams.

Conclusion: the usual stalemate where nobody wins, the conflict is never resolved, and the same conversation goes on for years.

Here's the thing: aren't you a bit tired of all the hassle? I get it - you are at that age where you feel rebellious, you want to stand up against the norms, you want to be independent and live your life your way. You've had enough of being treated like a kid and the lack of privacy. And your messy room isn't a dealbreaker for you. You hardly even notice it.

Reality check

If you are smart, you can avoid all these daily run-ins with your parents and still have your freedom and independence. In fact, by tidying up and cleaning your bedroom now and again, you will be one step closer to being treated the way you want. Instead of shooting yourself in the foot, which is what you are doing, you will get your parents off your back and enjoy your peace and quiet without arguments and ultimatums.

Does that make sense to you? OK, great. So, here are some suggestions on how to keep your bedroom organized (which you will benefit from) and keep your parents happy. It doesn't get any better than that!

Getting organized

As your room is your sanctuary, you would enjoy it more if it had that cool vibe, which you aren't going to get if it looks like a bomb has dropped. If I were you, I'd think about ways to keep on top of things so that it looks reasonably tidy. Not only will this make you feel more comfortable, but it will help you to be better organized. You don't need it to be perfect, just tidy and clean enough to pass the parent test.

- ### Set yourself a daily challenge

For a daily challenge, why not see if you can pick up ten things from the floor when you come home from school each day? Let's say, some socks, crisp wrappers, papers, books, jeans... whatever is lying around. It's amazing how much difference that can make if you keep it up.

- ### Know where things go

You've probably not realized that everything has its place. Rubbish goes in the rubbish bin, clothes go in closets and drawers, books go on your bookshelf or desk, and so on. If you have a small room and not much space, ask your parents to buy you some storage boxes and allocate each one for specific items. Label them if you need to - it can help!

- ### Set yourself a weekly challenge

How about doing ten things every week to keep your room ship-shape? You could change your sheets on your bed, for example, and put the dirty ones in the laundry basket in your bedroom or bathroom. Next, check under your bed if you dare... you won't find any monsters there but will very likely find that missing school book, takeaway pizza boxes, and dirty plates just waiting to attract ants or other pests.

- **Have a clearout**

Take a look at your desk and decide how much of it is clutter. Take any cups, glasses, or plates into the kitchen, and throw out any chewing gum and sweet wrappers that have been sitting there for a week or longer. Collect all of those mixed up handouts from school and put them in a folder that you can go through later.

- **Sort out your clothes**

You might hate doing this, and would much rather avoid it but hey, sooner or later you are going to run out of clean clothes. Apart from that, it's so time-consuming to have to rummage through the pile on your floor every time you are looking for those jeans or that T-shirt. If an item looks and smells clean, fold it and put it away. If it looks dirty or doesn't pass the smell test, put it in the wash. Easy!

- **Get rid of clutter**

Do you really need al those old Pokemon cards or Seventeen magazines? Is it necessary to hoard old clothes and shoes that you never wear? Just by going through a few items at a time, you will seriously reduce the amount of space all that stuff is taking up in your room.

Get some bin bags and fill them with anything that can be recycled. Find some local clothes banks where you can donate your old gear and you can even sell valuables online if you know how to do that.

- **There's a place for everything**

No matter how limited the space is in your room, you can create a place for all of your things and it's very simple:

- Books go on the bookcase
- Notebooks can go there too, or on your desk
- Jewelry can go in a jewelry box on your dresser

- Cosmetics can go in a small basket or container on your dresser
- Clothes go in the closet or drawers
- Stationary can go in pen holders, mugs, or boxes on your desk
- Shoes should go somewhere that you can't smell them like a shoe stand or even outside if they are protected from the weather
- Photos can go in frames or boxes

Where to store boxes

Once you have sorted your items into boxes or containers, you can label them if you like and keep them under your bed or in a cupboard. You don't need to have everything sprawled out across the floor or piled up next to your door like an obstacle course. Think more organization, more space.

- **Show off your prized possessions**

Remember those trophies you got for dancing or football? They've been hidden for so long behind other junk that you forgot to appreciate them. Now is the time to show them off. Clear your desk, book-shelf, dresser, or nightstand of all the other things you don't use, and let your special personal possessions take pride of place. Display those Star Wars figurines or glass ornaments given as gifts and enjoy your bedroom!

Tidying up your room isn't really that difficult if you break tasks down and do a bit at a time. As well as pleasing your parents, it also makes you appreciate what you have more. If you do want to claim your independence, there are plenty of other ways to earn that, and living in a dump isn't the best way to go about it.

Operation clean-up

The next thing you have to tackle is the actual cleaning, and that is definitely something you won't want to do. What's the point anyway, if it just gets dirty again? I understand your logic on this and I'm sure your parents feel exactly the same when they have to clean the rest of the house.

It's not my idea of fun either but someone needs to do it because, otherwise, dirt has a way of building up and is harder to get rid of the longer it stays there. How about doing some cleaning once a week or every two weeks? You can get your parents to help you and learn some nifty tips from them that save time and energy. Just ask them and I'm sure they'll be only too happy to lend a hand.

Some basic cleaning tasks can turn your bedroom into a place where you can hang out without worrying about mice wanting to take up residence there too.

- **Dust busting**

Believe it or not, dust is your number one enemy at the moment. I know it seems insignificant - you can hardly see it anyway. But it's there - lurking on every surface you touch and under every bed.

The problem with dust isn't that your mom hates it - that's normal. It's actually a combination of sloughed-off skin cells, hair, clothing fibers, bacteria, dust mites, bits of dead bugs, soil particles, pollen, and microscopic specks of plastic. Yuck!

Imagine breathing that in, day in, day out. Not a good thing to do, especially if you have allergies or suffer from a weak immune system. It can be a real health problem and is easily solved. You will find it on your desk, bookshelf, dresser, light fixtures, fans, and most other surfaces and you need to clean it the right way, starting from high up and working down.

You can vacuum the ceiling and floor with special attachments and use a damp cloth on other surfaces. Microfiber cloths are a good way to remove dust as it sticks to them while using a feather duster will just move it from one place to another. You can also use the microfiber cloth on your PC screen, TV, printer, or any other electrical appliance. Needless to say, you wouldn't use any damp cloth on anything electrical, and for safety, make sure you've unplugged it first.

- **Getting rid of dirt**

Your desk is probably teeming with disgusting microscopic bacteria that you can't see. It's where you eat, sneeze, and touch your face a lot when you are studying or using your PC - Gross, right? Wiping it down with a damp cloth or disinfectant wipes for surfaces takes literally ten seconds. While you're at it, you can wipe your nightstand, dresser, window sills, and any other surfaces in the room. It will smell great afterward!

- **Use the vacuum**

The vacuum cleaner is one of the first smart appliances ever invented and it's still a great way to clean your floor. Have you ever used one? It's quite easy - you just need to plug it in and press a button - not complicated at all for someone like you. Use it to get to those dust balls and food remnants under your bed and desk and you can even move furniture around to get into those hidden nooks and crannies.

You can use it no matter what your floor is made of - wood, tiles, marble, or plain carpet and there's also something called carpet cleaner that you sprinkle before you vacuum to get rid of strange smells.

The only downside to using vacuums is that the bag inside them can get full and will need changing often. You will know this is the case if it doesn't seem to be sucking things up and, depending on the make and model, you can buy refill bags at any hardware store. Your folks will be able to show you how to change the bag and you are ready to vax!

- **Mop away!**

If you have a floor without a carpet, it will need mopping. Make sure you've swept the floor first and collected any grunge in a dustpan before filling a bucket with soapy water and dipping the mop in. Wipe over the floor, rinsing the mop every few minutes as you go, beginning at the far side of the room until you reach the door. Ideally, you should do this once a week to get rid of stains like spilled coffee, milkshake, food, and dirt you carry in on your shoes. Take it from me - you will notice the difference!

We carry a lot of germs on our hands and then touch everything from light switches to door handles. Ask your parents to supply you with some disinfectant wipes you can use to clean fixtures on a regular basis and keep them on your desk so you don't forget to use them often.

- **Windows workout**

You may have a professional window cleaner who comes to your house every so often, especially if you live in a high apartment block, but they don't usually clean the insides. You can easily do it and all you need is some glass cleaner and window cloths.

Spray the glass and any mirrors in your room with the cleaner and wipe them in a circular motion until no streaks are left. You can remove any caked-in dirt or dust from the window tracks with an old toothbrush or all-purpose cloth.

Clean room, happy life

Cleaning doesn't take much time when you get into the swing of it and even though you might think you suck at it, practice makes perfect. It's a useful life skill to have for when you get older, especially if you plan on going away to college or living on your own.

For more motivation, putting on your favorite playlist while you do it will make each task a lot less painful. Otherwise, see it as a game and set yourself a time - if you finish it before the buzzer goes off, award yourself points. You can even try to beat your own record at vacuuming or dusting and treat yourself to a snack if you finish under the time limit.

The greatest benefit of cleaning your room, being tidier, and more organized, isn't that your mom and dad hassle you less, although that's a bonus. What you get is a sense of pride and satisfaction - you can look after yourself and still enjoy doing all the other things you want to. It doesn't mean you are a wimp or not cool when you have a tidy, ordered bedroom, nor that you've surrendered to the 'enemy'. It means you are acting freely, making your own choices, and becoming independent, which is what you want, right?

Some daily habits that might help you to keep tidying up time to a minimum are things like:

- Getting a laundry basket to put somewhere in your room so all dirty clothes can go directly in, instead of on the floor.
- Putting a small trash bin under your desk so you don't have to keep half-eaten apples or sweet wrappers
- Putting some hooks up on the back of your door for accessories like scarves, belts, or your school bag.
- Hanging your coat or jacket up when you enter your room after being out instead of throwing it on your bed.
- A tough one maybe - see if you can make your bed each morning. It will take you less than 2 minutes but look great when you return home from school later on in the day.

Now that you have mastered the art of maintaining a reasonably organized, clean, and tidy room, it could be a good idea to let your parents know that you will be responsible for keeping it that way from now on.

Explain to them that:

- they don't need to threaten you anymore with a reduced allowance or internet time.
- they don't need to go into your room to clean it when you aren't there.
- they don't need to invade your privacy or your personal space.
- they shouldn't expect perfection, even though you are doing your best.
- they don't need to bribe you to tidy up anymore. You've got this!

Like I said at the beginning of this chapter, being smart means avoiding arguments about the mess in your bedroom and how it stinks! By showing your parents that you are willing to tidy and clean it regularly, you will reduce those angry arguments and criticism. You can be cool, relax, chill out, and even find your school books easier, without shouting matches and threats.

I know you know it makes sense!

Top tips:

- *Arguments and rows with parents about the state of your bedroom can be avoided.*
- *You have to take responsibility for your own personal space.*
- *Being organized can make your life a lot easier.*
- *Challenging yourself to complete tasks is a great motivational tool.*
- *Cleaning is a useful life skill we can all learn to do.*
- *If you want privacy, freedom, and independence, show your folks your tidy bedroom!*

❧ 3 ❧
KITCHEN CLEANING -
MICROWAVES, DISHWASHERS
& THE ART OF DEFROSTING
THE FREEZER

I bet that the kitchen is your second favorite room in the house, after your bedroom. This is where you find food and also the place where you can dump your dirty dishes.

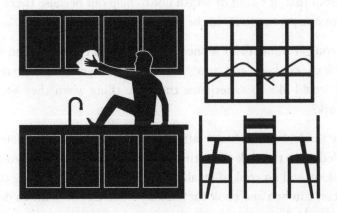

As long as your parents are there to shop, cook, and clean, the kitchen is the source of all happiness. But if they leave you home alone for a couple of days, would you be able to survive?

A lot of families raise their kids to be involved with kitchen tasks from an early age, and even four-year-olds can help with preparing food and loading the dishwasher, so what's your excuse? If you've never really been encouraged to help, then it's not easy to know how to use the oven, clear up after you, and basic hygiene tips. As for appliances like microwaves, fridges, and dishwashers, you might usually avoid them because they are 'far too complicated' to use.

If you are 13 and upwards, you belong to the digital generation and are most likely a whizz at anything high-tech. You can code, hack, understand computer lingo, and are totally wired into smart technology. You can access info at the swipe of a screen in seconds, spot a scammer a mile away, see through fake news immediately, and know how to use TikTok (I'm impressed)!

All of that, and you say a dishwasher is too complicated?

Luckily for you, I'm here to walk you through some of the skills that you really need to learn if you want to be able to feed yourself and avoid food poisoning when you eventually live alone.

You can always ask to help in the kitchen when your parents are around and I'm sure they will be pleased to see you taking an interest. Apart from that, it's kind of selfish not to help out because there is too much for one person to do in the kitchen.

When you get home from school or college, you expect to find everything clean, cooked, and ready for you. Did you know that your parents would like to experience the same thing when they get back from work?

Nobody wants to come home after a long day to find dirty plates and pans piled up in the sink or on the counters, grease and food droppings on the floor, and no cooked meal. Believe me, it's no fun having to take on a messy kitchen and cook for a family when all you want to do is to sit down and relax.

Now is a good chance to start picking up some kitchen skills and avoid any kitchen nightmares. We'll be taking a look at how to use basic appliances, including how to defrost a fridge/freezer, as well as learning a couple of kitchen cleaning basics, which you will earn bonus points for from your parents!

If you've got siblings, maybe you can arrange to share the tasks on a daily or weekly basis, but there's no harm in learning how things are done by yourself. All you need to do is roll up your sleeves and be ready to get your hands dirty.

How to use essential kitchen appliances

1. Microwave ovens

Microwaves are super convenient and use microwave radiation, which causes food molecules to vibrate at a high frequency, generating heat. It's so fast that you can warm up a plate of food in a few minutes. You can even use a microwave to make popcorn and heat up beverages like tea or coffee.

Regardless of the particular microwave model you have, the basic functions are generally the same for all ovens. Some also have a grill, to brown off meat, etc., while others are combis - allowing you the combination of heating and cooking at the same time. You can check the instructions that came with your model for more information.

Just place what you need heating up in the microwave and close the door. Select the settings you want and press the start button. Usually, food is heated up in 30-second bouts so if you need to warm up a steak, you will need to turn the dial or press the button a couple of times until you get to 3 or 4 minutes. Then, press start and wait for it to ping!

Did you know that you can also defrost food in a microwave? If you have a frozen chicken, for example, take off the wrapping and place it in a microwave-friendly dish. Pop the chicken in and select the defrost function, which usually goes by weight. If the chicken weighs 4lb, for example, select that weight and press the defrost function or dial, then start.

Microwave ovens heat up liquids much quicker than solids, so heating a cup of milk or coffee will only take seconds while a burger may take 2 to 3 minutes. You need to be careful when removing any liquids as they may splatter when you take them out and can cause serious skin burns.

You can cook most fruit and vegetables, melt butter, cheese, chocolate, make oatmeal, and even cook corn, potatoes, and fish in microwaves. Meat may take a while to cook and can dry up easily so you will need to keep an eye on it as time goes on.

After you have used the microwave and removed the food, wipe the inside down with a warm, damp cloth to remove any food that may have stuck to the inside.

Microwave dos and don'ts:

Only use microwave-safe dishes and plastic containers.

Don't try to cook pasta or anything that needs a lot of water.

Don't put aluminum foil, metal, plastic bags, paper bags, styrofoam, takeaway packaging, boiled eggs, or hot peppers in a microwave. They can all catch fire or explode!

Do arrange food evenly on the plate so it heats up consistently.

Do cover the dish to avoid splattering.

Do open the door frequently and stir carefully to distribute the heat.

Dishwashers

Everyone's best friend, dishwashers must be one of the greatest inventions ever! I don't know anyone who enjoys washing dirty dishes and fortunately, if you have a dishwasher, you don't need to. Despite what you might think, you don't have to be a mom to use it - you too have the superpower to load it, press the start button, and empty it when done.

There are different dishwasher models, but most have a top rack, a bottom rack, and a cutlery rack. If you aren't sure what goes where, you can ask your folks.

After you have eaten, take your plate and throw away any scraps before rinsing it under the kitchen tap. Place the plate in the dishwasher, making sure it's not overlapping with other plates already in there. You can also put in bowls, cups, mugs, glasses, plastic containers, dishwasher-safe baking trays, stainless steel pots & pans, spoons, knives, forks, and kitchen utensils. Place any knives with the blades facing down to avoid being stabbed when you take them out.

Regardless of which dishwasher you have, most detergent dispensers are on the bottom inside part of the dishwasher door. The detergent could be in tablet, liquid, or powder form, depending on what your parents are used to buying. Simply place whatever you have in the detergent dispenser and add any rinse aid to the rinse aid dispenser if there is one before closing the detergent door.

Close the dishwasher door and when it's full, select a wash cycle. You might be unsure about this if you've never done it before, so ask for help if you can't understand the symbols on the settings. Usually, though, there are at least three cycles - Quick, Normal, and Heavy Duty. Depending on your load and how dirty the dishes are, choose the cycle you think is the best by selecting one of the buttons usually located on the top of the dishwasher door. Press start and go!

The dishes will be warm when the cycle is finished, so leave them to cool down a bit before you open the door to use them.

3. Stove top and oven

The stove and oven are your answer to takeaway food! You might need mom or dad to supervise you if you aren't used to using them, as they can be dangerous. If you are older, you should still follow basic safety measures and never play with fire!

Your stove/oven will have temperature settings and you need to choose the correct one. If it runs on gas, you'll see a blue flame when you turn on one of the rings. If it works with electricity, you'll see the rings warming up with a red glow.

You may not be great at cooking and have no idea what you can or can't put in the oven, which pans to use, or how long something takes to cook. You can ask your parents, find recipes and instructions on the product packets, or watch YouTube videos to give you ideas.

If you want to use the oven, there are usually various control options such as bake, grill, convector fan only, etc. You also need to set the temperature gauge, which may show numbers like 1-10 (low to high), or degrees of heat (50°-250° F). Place food on the middle shelf if you want it to cook slowly and higher up if you want to grill it. The time it takes will depend on what you are cooking. Meat can take a couple of hours while a pizza will only need 30 minutes.

There are some safety basics you need to follow:

Whether a gas or electric stove, keep things like kitchen towels and utensils clear of the rings to stop them from burning.

Never leave anything you are cooking on the stove unattended.

Always make sure you have turned off the control knobs when you are done. An electric ring can stay hot for a while, even after it has been turned off.

Always use an oven glove to remove dishes from the oven, to avoid burning your hands.

4. Defrosting your freezer

The inside of your freezer shouldn't look like the polar arctic! If you can't pull out the trays or push them back in, and see a thick build-up of ice, then your freezer seriously needs defrosting. Some models do this job all by themselves but if you have an older or cheaper model, you have to do it manually. The more ice you see building up inside, the less space you have to store food and the less efficient the freezer is, so you need to defrost it every few months. You will need two-three hours for this but it's kind of fun when you actually get down to it.

First, remove all of the frozen food from the freezer to a cool location. If you can't use someone else's freezer for a while, fill up a cooler box with ice packs and place the food in there. Failing that, you can put the food in secured bags and store it somewhere cool - even outside if you live in a cold climate.

Next, turn off/unplug the freezer. If it's a fridge/freezer combo, the foodstuff will be fine in the fridge for a few hours, although you should avoid opening the door as much as possible to keep it chilled.

After that, get some old towels to place around the bottom of the freezer to soak up melting ice and excess water. Your freezer may have a drainage hose at the back so if it does, put the end of it in a low basin or bowl.

Remove all the shelves & drawers and leave the freezer door open. Some shelves may be stuck in ice, so be patient and wait for the big melt. You can use a kitchen spatula to scrape the surface ice into a bucket or basin and place a bowl of hot water in the freezer to speed up the process. You'll need to replace it every 10 minutes or so as it will get cold very quickly.

If you want to speed things up, use a hairdryer to melt the ice while you continue to scrape and collect it in a bowl as you go. Once you have melted all the ice, wipe the inside of the freezer with a warm cloth and leave it to dry for about 5 minutes with the door still open.

Then, place the trays and drawers back in, after washing them in warm, soapy water and drying them. When that's done, you can put all of the food back in, turn the freezer on or plug it in and you're done!

If any of the food has melted or thawed out, you probably need to throw it away as it could be inedible now. Don't risk cooking those frozen pizzas if they aren't frozen anymore - it could give you the runs, or worse.

Now that you've learned how to use these important kitchen appliances, how about upskilling and learning how to keep the kitchen clean and tidy? I know you may think that's not your job but you live and eat in the same house as everyone else, right?

It kind of is your shared responsibility, or at least you should know how to do the basics for when you go it alone in your own place.

If the kitchen isn't clean, it can be a serious health hazard and cooking is a lot easier when everything is in its right place. So, here are some tasks you should do regularly if you want to pass with a clean bill of health:

Wash dishes by hand. No need to wait for the dishwasher to do everything - just fill up the kitchen sink with warm soapy water and wash cups, plates, or anything else. Rinse them afterward in clean water to get rid of the soap suds and place them on a rack or kitchen towel to dry.

Clean the sink. A breeding ground for nasty bacteria, you should clean the sink every day with a dishcloth or sponge and some kitchen detergent. You can use chlorine, but wear rubber gloves and be sure to rinse the sink well with clean water when you are done.

Wipe down the counters, stove, microwave, and anything else to get rid of dried food, stains, dust, and bacteria you can't see. Again, use a mild kitchen cleaning agent, which you should find along with all the other house cleaning products.

Clear away any clutter into drawers and cupboards. Everything has its place in the kitchen and if you aren't sure what goes where, I'm sure your parents can help out with that.

Take out the trash. This may be the one job you know how to do, as it's been the extent of your chores so far. You also need to replace another clean trash bag in the garbage bin and find a container to use for recyclable waste if you don't already have one.

Sweep the kitchen floor. It collects a lot of dirt and grease so needs sweeping often, especially after you have just finished cooking. You can also mop it down but make sure not to step on it until it's dry to avoid slipping.

Clean the inside of the oven. Ideally, this should be done once a month so why not have a go? Some ovens are even self-cleaning, but if yours isn't, put on your rubber gloves and take out all of the oven racks. Spray the oven cleaner around the inside of your oven, including the back, sides, bottom, top, door, corners and crevices then close the oven and leave the spray to do its job. After that, take a damp cloth and wipe down the surfaces, collecting all the grunge and removing it. Go over the surfaces with a clean damp cloth and wash the racks with an abrasive sponge if needed. Dry them, and pop them back in the oven. Done!

Cleaning the fridge. There's nothing more gross than putting your hand in the fridge and grabbing a moldy apple or a chunk of green cheese so you need to have a clear-out now and again. Throw away any food that has passed its 'sell by' date and wipe the shelves and drawers with a warm soapy cloth before drying them off with a kitchen towel.

Cleaning the microwave. Ever noticed that the inside of your microwave smells funny? That's because food sticks to the sides and top when it's heating up and becomes a breeding ground for dangerous germs. Remove the turntable if it has one and wash it, then gently wipe the inside of the microwave with a warm, damp cloth before drying it with a clean kitchen towel. Remember to put the turntable back in its right place afterward.

You might not like the idea of having to get your hands dirty in the kitchen but believe me, when you are living on your own, nobody is going to be there to do it for you. Learn from the experts (your parents) while you have the chance and take the initiative to do things yourself instead of waiting for them to do everything.

It's not half as complicated as you imagine and you have no excuses now, so go for it and skill up!

Top tips:

- *Nobody enjoys kitchen duty, but we've all got to eat!*
- *Microwaves are cool, if you know how to use them,*
- *Learning how to use the dishwasher will take you two minutes.*
- *Your stovetop and oven are there to cook meals, so use them.*
- *Your freezer needs to be defrosted if you want to fit anything in it.*
- *Keeping the kitchen clean will keep you out of the hospital.*

HOW TO BUDGET, BUY GOOD FOOD, AND COOK IT

S ooner or later, you are going to have to learn how to handle your money, buy food, and cook it. It's a part of life and unless you intend to live on takeaway food for life and end up penniless, there's no getting out of it.

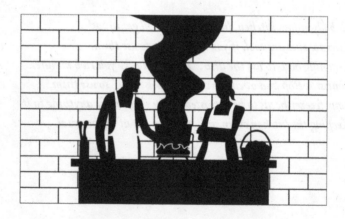

You might have no idea how to budget and don't know how much money your parents spend each month on groceries.

As teens, we are lucky, food either magically turns up on the table or arrives inside a delivery box. In real life though, people actually go to the supermarket, try to spend only what they can afford, and buy food-stuff that can make wholesome, healthy meals.

You might be surprised at how expensive some food items can be. And if you haven't got a clue how to check if something is fresh, or how to plan a weekly menu, then this chapter is for you.

When you go to the supermarket, grocery store, or farmer's market with a certain amount of money in your pocket, you have to make sound choices on what to buy based on your needs. You can blow it all on tubs of Ben and Jerry's ice cream, potato chips, and Coca-Cola, but then, what will you eat for the rest of the week?

Budget buying

By learning how to spend wisely now, you will never starve, and the sooner you learn how to do that, the easier it will become. Budgeting is useful in every aspect of life and it all starts at home. The next time your folks go grocery shopping, tag along with them and ask how much they want to spend.

Note what they are buying and how quickly the cart soon fills up with items you might never have thought of buying yourself. Then, see what their total bill is and check if they remained on budget or not. Most likely, they will. This is because they have a very good idea of what they need to feed the family and will resist buying unnecessary products that can make them go over budget.

Now it's your turn. Let's imagine that you are living on an allowance or earning your own money. How much of it are you going to allocate to your weekly grocery shopping? What else are you going to spend it on? (Don't say fast food - that's the wrong answer! Lol) You have to consider things like:

- What other expenses you have, such as rent and electricity/gas bills
- How much you need to pay for the wifi and your mobile contract.
- How much money you need to go out with friends

- How much money you need for personal items such as shaving cream or shampoo
- How much you should put to one side for unexpected expenses

When it comes to groceries, you might not know how much money you need until you get to the supermarket or stores. Set yourself a reasonable amount and then make a shopping list before you leave home.

Check in the cupboards, pantry, and fridge to see what you need, which could include everything from dried ingredients like rice to meat, fruit & vegetables, and dairy products like milk & cheese. You should also plan ahead for what meals you can make over the next seven days and I'll give you some recipe options a bit later.

Once you have made a grocery list, you should try to stick to it instead of being tempted into buying non-essentials, which will eat away at your budget.

Armed with your shopping list, hit the supermarket aisles and take the time to look at each product. When you are trying to decide what to buy, here are some things to take into account:

- Compare prices of premium brands vs. cheaper/store brands.
- Check the 'use by' dates, especially on things like milk and bread.
- Compare unit prices (e.g. $1.50 per 100g for a smaller pack vs. $1.20 per 100g for a larger pack of the same item).
- Check the nutritional information on packaging and see if it contains anything you may be allergic to or have an intolerance for, such as nuts or gluten.
- '3 for the price of 2' promotions might seem like a bargain, but don't buy them if you only need one item.
- Calculate how much you are spending in your head or on your phone as you go along.
- Ask for a free membership/loyalty card that offers bonus

points or vouchers you can use at the checkout when you have collected enough of them.

- Look out for reduced products which need to be sold 'today', such as fresh pasta or marinated chicken wings. You'll usually find these marked down in price toward supermarket closing time so the later you go shopping, the better.
- Supermarkets are generally cheaper than your corner store and better than online grocery shopping, as you can't see what is fresh and what isn't.
- Basic foodstuffs like pasta, rice, flour, eggs, and canned tomatoes are always good things to have in your kitchen cupboards and are relatively cheap to buy in any store.

How to tell what is fresh

You should check the 'sell by' and 'use by' date of everything you buy in the supermarket, which will be written somewhere on the packaging. Even frozen and dried foods have their limits, so it's a good idea to make sure to check everything you put into your cart. You probably find it hard to know just how fresh or ripe some things are, so here's a quick guide:

Don't buy any jars, cans, cartons, or bottles that look bloated or damaged, such as mayonnaise, fresh milk, or beans.

Vegetables are tricky.

I've listed a few common ones for you to look out for:

Potatoes - Don't buy potatoes that are green or sprouting.

Onions - Don't buy onions that are soft or oozing.

Carrots - Don't buy carrots that seem floppy, and aren't bright orange.

Cucumbers - Don't buy cucumbers if they aren't hard and haven't got a deep green color.

Eggplants/Aubergines - These should have a light purple color and be firm to the touch.

Cauliflower and broccoli - Don't buy them if they have black spots or feel soft.

Mushrooms - Only buy mushrooms that have their caps attached to the stem and have a clear, blemish-free color.

Frozen veggies are a great alternative if you want to be on the safe side.

Fresh fruit.

You can usually tell just by looking at fruit how fresh it is but if you aren't sure, here are some tips:

Fruit should have a bright, vibrant color - cherries look red, oranges look orange, and so on.

Bananas - Ripe bananas are yellow but it's OK if they have some speckled brown spots on them. You can buy ones that are still slightly green and leave them to ripen. Don't put bananas in the fridge, they don't like it.

Apples - Whether red or green, check they aren't bruised or too soft.

Watermelons - Watermelon slices should look deep red and if you buy a whole one, it's OK if it has some yellow areas on the outer skin. One way to check if a watermelon is ripe is to slap it to see if it makes a hollow sound.

Melons - Melons should smell sweet and feel firm. You will know they are ready to eat if you press the top or bottom with your fingers and they feel spongy but not too soft.

Pineapples - Ripe pineapples will have a sweet smell, especially near the stem, and without any dark spots on the skin.

Plums - Plums should feel a little bit spongy when you squeeze them and have a deep color.

Strawberries - Strawberries ripen and go off very quickly so choose firm ones with a bright color. They should also smell sweet.

Oranges & Lemons - Fresh oranges and lemons have a vibrant citrus smell and are firm to the touch.

Avocados - Check that the skin is a deep green color and not bruised. Ripe avocados should feel firm but not rock hard or too soggy.

Tomatoes - Technically a fruit, tomatoes should be firm, have a bright color, without any damage to the skin,

If you prefer, you can buy dried fruit such as dates, mango, banana, and pineapple.

Meat.

As well as checking that the meat counter looks clean and organized, focus on the color of the meat you want to buy. It should range from pinkish to pale red and not brown. If you want to buy minced meat, ask the butcher to select a cut and ground it there and then for you.

Eggs.

Check the stamp on each egg, which shows you two dates: the 'sell by' date and the 'use by' date. If they have expired, don't buy them.

Fish.

Fresh fish will NOT smell fishy or overpowering. The eyes will be bright, the gills red, and if you can touch the fish, it should feel firm when you press it and flexible.

Bread.

Supermarket bread might have been on the shelf for a few days so check to see if it still feels crisp but not hard. Otherwise, trust your local bakery to have fresh bread just out of the oven.

Meat Free.

Vegetarian and vegan food is freely available nowadays. Some meat-free products such as veggie sausages and burgers can taste as good (or even better) than the originals. Store these in the fridge or freezer. There are now lots of vegetarian or vegan food available in supermarkets.

Time to cook!

Once you have done your grocery shopping, it's time to think about what meals you can cook. You may be a maestro at microwave meals but haven't tried to cook anything more adventurous than pot noodles (or ramen noodles). If you are not old enough to cook unsupervised, make sure you have an adult there to help you at all times.

Here are some quick and easy recipes that won't break your bank balance and if what you make tastes good, eat it!

BREAKFAST/SNACKS

Scrambled eggs

Crack 2 or 3 eggs into a bowl. Add a little milk, cream, or sour cream.

Beat the eggs with a fork or hand whisk. Heat a flat, non-stick pan over a medium-low heat and add a knob of butter.

After it's melted, pour in the eggs and keep them moving around the pan with a spatula or wooden spoon.

When the eggs look almost done, turn off the heat and add salt and pepper. You can also add grated cheese if you like. Serve and enjoy!

Banana oatmeal

Put half a cup of oatmeal in a small pan with one ripe, spotty banana. Add half a cup of water, half a cup of milk, some cinnamon, and a pinch of salt.

Cook over a low heat, stirring and mashing the banana with a wooden spoon. Keep stirring for 8 to 10 minutes.

Take the oatmeal off the heat to thicken a little more, then scoop into a bowl. You can add chopped walnuts or blueberries if you like. Done!

Homemade pancakes

- Crack two eggs into a large bowl and add 2 tablespoons of sugar, 2 tablespoons of butter, and half a cup of milk. Mix the ingredients together with a fork or hand whisk.
- Slowly stir in 1 cup of flour, 1 teaspoon of baking powder, and a pinch of salt. The mixture should have the consistency of fresh cream when you are finished.
- Heat up a small skillet or flat pan and melt a knob of butter

until it starts bubbling. Slowly pour in enough pancake batter to make the pancake size you prefer, flipping it with a spatula after one minute.

- Serve and add your favorite toppings, such as maple syrup, honey, ice cream, yogurt or fresh berries. Delicious!

LUNCH/DINNER

Baked (jacket) potatoes

- Scrub the skins of a couple of medium-sized potatoes until clean and prick them with a fork. Wrap them in aluminum foil and place in the oven on a baking tray. Set the temperature to about 400°F (200°C) and leave them to bake for 1 hour.
- Check to see if the potatoes are done by prodding them with a fork. When they feel soft inside, take them out of the oven and leave to cool.
- For toppings, you can mix some grated carrot and white cabbage in a bowl with mayonnaise to make coleslaw. You can also use tuna with mayo or cooked bacon bits with grated cheese. It's up to you what topping to add, depending on what is handy.

How to cook pasta:

Half-fill a large pan with water and bring to the boil. Add the pasta and check the packet for cooking times (spaghetti might need 8 to 9 minutes, while rigatoni might need 10). When done, turn off the heat and drain the pasta in a colander over the sink. Place it back in the pan and swish it around with a teaspoon of olive oil before serving.

Spaghetti sauce

Heat 2 tablespoons of olive oil in a large skillet on a medium-high heat. Add 1 lb of ground beef and let it brown slightly, stirring all the time. Add half a cup of diced onion, 1 crushed garlic clove, 1 can of crushed tomatoes, 1 teaspoon of oregano, some freshly chopped basil, and salt & pepper.

Leave the sauce to simmer, stirring occasionally, and add a little water if it seems too thick or is sticking to the bottom of the pan. Cook for about half an hour and serve over spaghetti or pasta of your choice.

Mac and Cheese

Turn the oven on to 400°F (200°C) and grease a medium-sized casserole dish (9x13-inch) with a knob of butter. Half-fill a large pan with salted water and when it is boiling, add a packet of elbow (Gomiti) pasta. When it's cooked (about 10 minutes), drain and leave to one side in the heated casserole dish.

Meanwhile, melt 5 tablespoons of butter on a low heat in a large pan and slowly whisk in 5 tablespoons of all-purpose flour. Mix into a smooth paste then pour in 2 cups of warm milk, stirring until the sauce thickens.

Take off the heat and add 2 cups of grated cheese (try a mix of cheddar & mozzarella), a dash of mustard powder, and a pinch of salt.

Pour over the pasta and cook in the oven until bubbly and golden brown (about 15-20 minutes), then serve.

Chicken fajitas

Mix half a teaspoon of chili powder, 1 tablespoon of cumin, one crushed garlic clove, 1 teaspoon of paprika, 1 teaspoon of oregano, and a touch of salt and pepper in a large bowl.

Take 4 chicken breasts and cut them into large, long strips on a chopping board. Toss them in the spice mix in the bowl, making sure they are completely coated. Put a few tablespoons of olive oil in a large skillet and add the chicken, cooking it on a medium to medium-high heat for about 10-15 minutes.

Add sliced red, green, or yellow bell peppers and onions to the pan and sauté until cooked properly. Squeeze the juice of half a lime or lemon over everything and serve the fajitas with tortillas, sour cream, avocado, and any other tasty topping.

DESSERT

Peanut butter treats

Add a quarter of a cup of butter to a large heatproof bowl, along with 1 bag or 5 cups of mini marshmallows. Microwave for one-minute intervals on medium power, stirring now and then until they are both melted.

Stir half a cup of peanut butter into the bowl and 6 cups of corn flakes or rice crispies. Press the gooey mixture into a flat baking tray and leave it to set.

You can pour melted chocolate over the top if you like and cut the treat into bite-sized slices when the chocolate has cooled and hardened. Delicious!

Chocolate pudding

Preheat the oven to 350°F (180°C) and combine 1 cup of flour, 1 teaspoon of baking powder, half a cup of sugar, 1 tablespoon of cocoa, and a pinch of salt in a large mixing bowl.

Stir in 2 tablespoons of melted butter, half a cup of milk, and 1 teaspoon of vanilla. Mix well with a large wooden spoon until thick and clumpy.

Spread the mixture into a greased, medium-sized casserole dish and leave it to one side.

In another bowl, mix together a quarter of a cup of brown sugar, a quarter of a teaspoon of salt, and 1 tablespoon of cocoa. Sprinkle over the pudding mix and carefully pour 1 cup of boiling water on top.

Bake in the oven for 30 minutes, or until the top is almost set. Serve it warm with your favorite ice cream. Finger-licking good!

Fruit Fantastic

Take 3 or 4 apples, pears, or peaches and peel the skins. Chop into large pieces and remove the cores or stones.

Place in a medium-sized pan, add a dash of lemon juice, 4 tablespoons of water, 1 tablespoon of brown sugar, and cook on a low heat for 3 to 4 minutes.

When the fruit has softened, add a sprinkle of cinnamon and serve in a dessert bowl with Greek yogurt. Easy!

There are plenty more recipes out there for you to discover and as long as you use fresh ingredients, you should get great results every time. I've started you off with simple meals that you are probably familiar with before you try out anything fancy that you've never eaten before.

You don't need expensive kitchen equipment to cook. A few pots and baking dishes, a mixing bowl and hand whisk, a wooden spoon and spatula, as well as a reasonably good knife and chopping board, are sufficient for now.

Try to prepare and cook food BEFORE you get hungry, otherwise, you will end up ordering a takeaway, which isn't half as nutritious. You will also save money by cooking your own meals and enjoy them much more than if someone else had made them for you.

Another good thing about cooking yourself is that you can adapt everything to your specific dietary requirements. You may be a vegan or vegetarian, have allergies to nuts, be lactose intolerant, or need gluten-free ingredients, so cooking yourself gives you absolute control over what goes into your body.

When you cook for one, you really don't want to waste anything and, fortunately, you don't have to. Most food can be saved for one or two days and you can even cook double the amount you need if you want to avoid cooking every day. Pop half of it into a sealed container when cooked and after it's cooled down, store in the fridge, ready to be heated up in the microwave when you are next hungry.

Get inspired by watching your favorite YouTube chefs and ask parents, relatives or friends for their favorite recipes. Once you get the hang of the basics, you can experiment more with different ingredients and you might even discover your hidden culinary talents.

You'll definitely find out that cooking isn't a chore: it's a fun, creative way to make delicious home-cooked meals on a budget and eat like royalty!

Try it and see for yourself!

Top tips:

- *Learning how to stick to a budget and shop wisely is a survival skill.*
- *Only buy what you need, armed with a shopping list and a calculator.*
- *Check out the cheapest places to shop where you can find the freshest produce.*
- *Never buy anything that doesn't seem fresh as it is a waste of money and a potential health risk.*
- *Start by cooking familiar dishes that you like before experimenting with more complicated recipes.*
- *Shopping for food and cooking your own meals is an economical, healthy habit that will serve you well in life.*

❧ 5 ❧
SMELLY SOCKS AND STINKY ARMPITS - TEENS AND PERSONAL HYGIENE

Are you living up to the stereotype of being a smelly teenager with bad breath, sweaty armpits, and stinky socks?

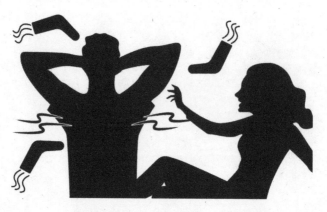

Great — make the most of it now because you won't get away with it when you are older!

Young people from pre-teen upwards are well-known for going through different phases, and that's part of growing up. You might suddenly decide to stop taking showers or not worry about having greasy hair that covers your face.

Personal hygiene may not be high on your list at the moment and you don't care if your feet smell. Even if your parents nag you about it from noon till night, it's not going to make you change your bad habits. I know: you have better things to do than taking a shower, like playing video games or chatting with friends. Maybe you intend to do it later, but then it always gets too late and you can't be bothered.

I get that you want to assert your independence and your parents probably don't realize that their comments are annoying and even sound like criticism. What's it to them if you want to skip having a shower after all? Their nagging might also make you feel even more determined to ignore them or go against their advice because nobody likes being told what to do.

You are right. It's up to you how you treat your body as you grow, but I'm going to drop a WARNING here: poor personal hygiene can be seriously bad for your health, not to mention your social life.

With all of the hormonal changes going on in your body, you've probably noticed that you sweat more, have outbreaks of acne, and are growing hair in very personal places. All of that is normal but it doesn't mean you have to stop washing. In fact, cleanliness is more important now than when you were a kid. Back then, you probably relied on your parents to look after you, but now, you are fully capable of doing that yourself. The thing is, you might not be aware of what problems you could face health-wise if you don't start taking more care of your hygiene habits.

It's not just another excuse for your folks to have a go at you, even though it may feel that way. Acne or infected spots now can leave permanent scarring if you don't take care of them. Sweating under the armpits can cause chaffing and other annoying irritations if you don't shower often enough.

Not brushing your teeth daily can lead to gum infections, tooth decay, and bad breath. It's not a pretty picture, so looking after your health begins here.

On a social level, even your best friend may feel uncomfortable telling you that you have a body odor issue so even if they don't mention it, that doesn't mean that they haven't noticed. I'm sure you've also noticed that some of your friends don't exactly smell like a bed of roses, but you would never dream of mentioning it to them.

If you are a guy, believe me, girls don't find overpowering sweaty smells that appealing. There's a difference between having a healthy after-workout odor and smelling like a trash can. If you are a girl, I can guarantee you that boys aren't attracted to breath that smells like fermented French cheese, no matter how much lip gloss you wear.

Looking after your personal hygiene may seem like one more chore you have to do, but you aren't doing it for anyone else. It's in your best interests at the end of the day and all your parents are doing is trying to keep you healthy, which is their job. I really don't think you need me to tell you how important it is to feel fresh, clean, and practice self-care.

If it's the case that you don't have anyone to show you the basics, like a responsible adult or older sibling, this chapter will tell you all you need to know. Once you start getting into a healthy hygiene routine, it's something you'll do without even thinking about it and will feel the benefits immediately.

There are some personal hygiene basics you need to follow regularly and most of them take very little time. Here's the list of must-do's that you need to start applying:

- Brush your teeth twice a day and floss after every meal if you can.
- Shower or bathe when you need to, which may mean every day or every second day.
- Use deodorant or antiperspirant.
- Wash your face regularly.
- Wash your hair regularly.
- Trim your nails when needed.
- Wear clean socks and underwear every day.

Now, let's take a look at each one to find out why it is so important.

- **Dental Hygiene**

When you brush your teeth frequently, think about how much better your breath will smell. If that's not enough incentive for you, imagine how much money you will save in the future on dental procedures. It's not just your teeth you are looking after though. Apart from removing harmful bacteria that builds up and causes tooth decay, your gums will also benefit.

A lot of people suffer from gum disease, the most common one being gingivitis, which makes your gums recede over time, and can lead to a loss of teeth if you leave it too long. Ideally, you should brush your teeth after each meal but if not, at least once a day. Flossing is also really useful because it gets into those tight spaces your toothbrush can't reach and helps to remove any nasty bacteria lurking there.

Did you know? The sugar in soda, sugary drinks, or sports drinks creates bacteria called plaque, which eats away at the enamel protecting your teeth. It also makes your breath smell gross.

- **Showering and Taking A Bath**

Showering after doing any sport or exercise is a hygiene law that you can't afford to ignore. But even if you don't play soccer, softball, tennis, work out, or do exercise, regular showers or taking baths should be on the top of your self-care list.

You don't need to shower or bathe every day but definitely every second day, especially now that your body is secreting so much sweat. It's best to use a mild shower gel or soap so that you aren't stripping your skin of its natural body oils.

A few minutes in the shower is enough, as long as you reach the parts that need it more, such as your underarms, groin/private parts, bottom, and in between your toes. Showers use less water than having a bath but if you prefer that, don't soak for too long, and be sure to rinse the soap suds off afterward.

Did you know? 5 to 10 minutes is enough time to get clean in the shower. Short, lukewarm showers are better if you have dry skin or eczema and it's a good idea to use a body moisturizer afterward, depending on your skin type.

- **Deodorant and antiperspirant**

What's the difference and why should you use them? Both are a personal choice, but it's a good idea to use either if you don't pass the sniff test - just smell your armpits and decide! Deodorants mask the smell of sweat while antiperspirants are supposed to block the sweat glands altogether, which can lead to painful lumps if you overuse them.

If you want to avoid using chemicals, there are plenty of products out there with natural ingredients. Some of them may smell nice, while others are odorless, and it's up to you which one you go for. If you shave your underarms, make sure to use deodorant for sensitive skin to avoid irritation.

Did you know? It's not necessarily your sweat that smells. It's the bacteria on your skin breaking down the sweat that produces an odor. The damp warmth of your armpits is an ideal environment for that bacteria to breed.

- **Washing your face**

A dirty face doesn't cause acne - that happens because your sebaceous glands are producing more oil in the pores of your skin, which can get trapped. But not washing your face enough doesn't help the situation as it's exposed to dirt, sweat, oil, and even make-up on a daily basis. You should have a 3-step skincare routine, regardless of your gender, and make sure you stick to it.

First, use a gentle face wash on your skin or ask at the pharmacy for a medicated face wash for acne. Secondly, wash your face gently, without scrubbing or using rough cloths, and rinse off any face wash very well. Thirdly, pat dry with a soft, clean towel and only use a moisturizer that is oil-free and preferably at least a 15 SPF.

Did you know? To prevent acne from spreading, you should wash your hands before and after touching your face, clean your cell phone often with a disinfectant wipe, change your pillowcase frequently, and drink plenty of water.

- **Washing your hair**

As you go through adolescence, which means bodily changes as you grow from child to adult, your hormones go into overdrive. One of the results is an excess of oil produced by the sebaceous glands. You'll notice this the most in your skin, hair, and scalp. Each strand of hair has its own sebaceous (oil) gland, which keeps it shiny and waterproof, but the excess oil can make your hair look greasy and limp. You need to keep on top of this with regular shampooing, be that every day or at least every other day.

There are hundreds of brands for you to choose from in your local drugstore but it's a good idea to select one specifically for oily hair. Use warm water and just a small amount of shampoo to work up a lather and don't scrub too hard as this can irritate your scalp. You might want to avoid using a conditioner afterward because it can leave your hair feeling heavy although there are products available for oily hair.

Did you know? You might like using hair styling products such as wax, mousse, or gel but these can make your hair feel super greasy. Look out for products that say 'greaseless' or 'oil-free' and use them sparingly.

- **Nail care**

If you are a girl, you may already look after your nails and like to style them with different nail polishes, while most boys don't pay attention to their nails at all. Whatever the case, your fingernails are the perfect breeding ground for germs, which can then pass into your mouth when you eat with your hands. The germs can also spread to any part of your body that you touch, and we all know the importance of keeping our hands clean.

Ideally, you should scrub your nails with a nail brush when you wash your hands. Apart from that, keeping them short prevents dirt from getting trapped underneath them and stops you from biting them. You can use a nail clipper or scissors on your hands and if you prefer your nails long, make sure to keep them clean. Don't forget your toenails too, which can also harbor dirt and cause smelly feet.

Did you know? Your toenails should be clipped straight across to prevent the corner or side from growing into the soft flesh. This can cause pain, redness, swelling, and an ingrown toenail, which might need to be surgically removed if it gets too bad.

- **Clean socks and underwear**

Your clothes soak up sweat like a sponge so you need to change them often and wear clean ones, especially underwear and socks. These collect all the dead skin cells, sweat, and bodily fluids you give off and bacteria love to grow there, creating quite a stink!

These nasty microbes can also cause skin rashes in places you really don't want and if left to fester, can have serious consequences such as bladder cancer or even kidney failure.

Clean underwear is non-negotiable and if you don't have that many boxer pants or comfy undies, you can wash them by hand with a mild detergent as soon as you change them and let them dry in the sun. The same goes for socks, which soak up sweat and create a warm, dark environment for fungus to grow that can cause athlete's foot and ringworm.

Did you know? Cotton underwear and socks are much better for your skin than synthetic materials as they allow the pores to breathe. A lot of fashion underwear is made up mostly of nylon, which can make you sweat and itch more, so it's best to avoid wearing them if you can.

Those are the basic self-care habits you should get used to doing regularly. They will make you feel a lot better about yourself and even improve your self-confidence. No more hiding behind that greasy hair from now on!

There are some other hygiene tips I want to give you that I'm sure you will find useful. Not all of them may apply to you, but maybe you have a friend who could benefit from them, so let's take a look.

Shaving and hair removal

- From the age of 13 onward (and sometimes even younger), you start to enter adulthood, and one of the changes involves hair growth on your legs, underarms, private areas, and face. Learning how to shave any of these areas isn't easy, and you should get a trusted adult to help you until you get the hang of it.
- If you are intending to use razors or electric razors, you need to be very careful to avoid cutting yourself and use enough soap or shaving cream to reduce irritation.
- There are many kinds of hair removal products on the market such as wax and depilatory creams. Ask an adult or expert before you use anything on your skin, even if friends tell you it was OK for them. Everyone's skin is different.
- Shaving is a personal choice and isn't related to cleanliness. You can have underarm hair and still be clean, just as you can grow a facial beard. You may feel pressured to shave leg or arm hair but need to consider this before you start and make sure you are doing it for the right reasons.

Grooming

- Keeping yourself clean and tidy is a basic essential and you can also pay attention to your overall appearance by visiting a beauty salon or men's barber.
- Keep your hair tidy with regular visits to the hairdressers, pluck your eyebrows or have them done by an eyebrow specialist, and use skincare products that compliment you.
- Take care of your clothes, washing them regularly and ironing

them before you wear them if needed. In general, taking pride in the way you look will help you feel more ready to face the world and even make others more comfortable around you.

Menstruation

- You should know that girls begin menstruating at some point in their teens. The monthly menstrual cycle, or periods, as it is often called, is a series of hormonal or physical changes that prepare a woman's body for pregnancy. If the pregnancy doesn't take place, the body resets until next month, during which time blood is shed from the uterus and through the vagina.
- For girls menstruating, proper hygiene is extremely important. You will definitely need adult help to select the best sanitary products for you once you begin and can choose from products like tampons, sanitary pads, and menstrual cups.
- It's also crucial to shower regularly, practice proper hygiene when using sanitary products, and change your underwear as often as necessary. Please be sure to ask your mother or female relatives for any help and support.

Busting teenage myths about hygiene

You might talk a lot with your friends about certain aspects of personal hygiene, and not always have the facts. There's a lot of misinformation out there and some myths that need to be busted. Here are a few common ones that you may have heard of:

- **Greasy food causes acne.** No, it doesn't. Acne is caused by overactive sebaceous glands that kick off when you are going through adolescence and it isn't linked to what you eat. Having said that, it's not a bad idea to cut down on greasy food as it can make you overweight if you eat too much of it.
- **Getting a suntan will cure acne.** It would be nice if this were true, but it isn't. Whiteheads, blackheads, lesions, and other forms of acne that usually look red can temporarily fade

while you are in the sun, but your skin is actually being dried of oil. This causes your body to compensate for that by producing even more oil, which means that there's a higher chance of having another acne breakout later on.

- **Shaving makes hair grow back faster and thicker.** Like it or not, this just isn't true. Shaving your hair doesn't change its thickness, color, or rate of growth. It does give it a blunt tip, which may feel coarser and seem thicker, although in reality it isn't.
- **Masturbation causes blindness, madness, and other terrible calamities.** You may be pleased to hear that masturbation is totally harmless and is a natural expression of sexuality for both men and women of all ages. It doesn't cause any physical injury or harm to the body, although some cultures and religions oppose masturbation or label it as sinful, which can lead to feelings of shame and guilt.

And on that note, I hope that you've picked up some useful information here about how to practice more self-care. Hopefully, you have also gained a better understanding of why personal hygiene is important. You should always ask an adult you trust when you are unsure about any aspects of your health and seek medical help if needed.

Take care of your body and enjoy your teenage years, because they pass by very quickly!

Top tips:

- *You can be a rebellious teenager and still take showers and wear clean clothes.*
- *Brushing your teeth daily prevents bad breath and gum disease.*
- *Taking a shower or bath often reduces nasty body odors, especially after doing sports or exercise.*
- *Deodorants and antiperspirants are useful when you want to mask body smells.*
- *Washing your hair and face regularly prevents acne from spreading and removes excess oil from your skin and hair.*

- *Keep your nails short and if you prefer them long, scrub them well to get rid of bacteria.*
- *Wearing clean socks and underwear prevents bacteria and fungus from growing.*
- *Don't believe all the stories your friends tell you about health and hygiene - a lot of it is untrue.*

✤ 6 ✤

LOOKING AFTER YOUR CAR

Congratulations! You've recently passed your driving test and now have wheels! There's nothing cooler than rolling into school or picking up your friends in your new vehicle, especially if it's a super slick model. Freedom is yours, at last!

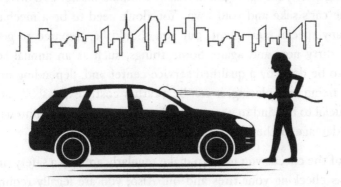

Owning your first car can give you a big buzz as the road of life stretches out before you. Of course, you need to gain more confidence with your driving skills but from here on in, everything is sweet. You don't have to depend on your folks now to drive you around, your friends will be impressed, and that amazing sense of independence is a game-changer.

Owning a car is an exciting initiation into the adult world and along with it comes quite a bit of responsibility. First of all, you have to pay for the gas, although you might get help with that from your parents or use part of your allowance. They may also pay for all of the other things like insurance and road tax, but expect you to contribute and take it to the car wash or clean it yourself.

There's a lot of joy to be had looking after your first car and even if it is second-hand, you will still want it to shine and look great. If you have any interest in cars, you will know that they also need regular mainte-nance. You may already know what's needed to keep your motor healthy and running, and be keen to learn more.

On the other hand, you might have no idea whatsoever and aren't particularly interested in learning about what goes on under the bonnet. If that's the case, you should really learn some basics for your own good. Knowing how to change a tire, for example, can be crucial if you get a flat one in the middle of nowhere.

Looking after your car is a skill that you should master as a driver, both for the car's sake and your own. You don't need to be a mechanic or have any special equipment, but you should be prepared to get your hands dirty now and again. Some things, such as an annual service, need to be done by a qualified service center and, depending on what needs fixing or replacing, it can be a rather costly expense. That's why it's crucial to be kind to your car and stay on top of any maintenance to avoid damage further down the line.

A lot of the checks you need to make regularly are also a safety priority, such as checking your tires and oil. Also, you are legally required to ensure that certain things are working correctly, such as taillights. If not, you could receive a heavy fine when stopped by traffic police. As well as that, there are certain things you should always carry with you in your car, such as jump leads/cables and a first aid kit.

You can take a look at your car user manual if you have one, which will help you to familiarize yourself with what goes where. Nowadays, you can download these online from the car manufacturer. If you are feeling adventurous enough, you can enroll in a car maintenance workshop, where you'll get hands-on advice and practical tips from your instructor. Otherwise, ask a family member or friend who is used to cars to help you understand how everything works and where each car part is.

First, let's go through some of the basic car maintenance checks that anyone can do. Before you do anything on your car, make sure you always have a car tool kit with you, which you can store in the trunk.

Basic maintenance tasks

1. **Keep your car clean inside and out**

- Taking your car for a regular wash helps to protect the paint and gives you the chance to check for any scratches or damage to the bodywork of the car.
- If you want to clean the car yourself, you will need items like sponges, a bucket, car-cleaning shampoo, and wax or polish.
- Obviously, you need to keep your windows clean so you can see out of them and should use special glass-cleaning products for this. Make sure you also clean your headlights because dirt can make them appear dim and prevent you from seeing and being seen when driving at night.
- Use a hand-held vacuum cleaner to pick up dirt inside the car and special spray polish for the dashboard or a damp cloth.
- Keep all those nobs, vents, and switches free of dust and throw out any rubbish such as paper or coffee cups that you don't need.
- Keep your car tidy by storing items in the special compartments that come with your particular model.

1. **Check the tire pressure and tread wear**

- Your car tires need to have a certain pressure to make them safe when you are on the road. Tire pressure is measured as PSI(pounds per square inch) and the correct pressure is crucial to your safety. Under-inflated tires can overheat and wear unevenly, while over-inflated tires can blow out.

- Your manufacturer will tell you what the tire pressure should be for your model or you can find it on a sticker inside the driver's side door. The recommended pressure can range between 30 and 35 PSI but you need to check it to be sure.
- If you don't have a tire pressure gauge, you'll find them at your local gas station and can ask the attendant to help you. Otherwise, you can buy your own and choose from three different types:

(i) **Pen-type pressure gauge.** These have a ruler-like rod that slides in and out of a sleeve to measure air pressure.

(ii) **Dial pressure gauge.** This has a numbered dial with a watch-like hand.

(iii) **Digital pressure gauge.** This displays numbers on a digital screen.

- To use a pressure gauge, remove the tire valve cap. Make sure the gauge is evenly pressed into the valve stem after you have taken the cap off. Push on the gauge until you get a reading and check what number comes up. Remove the pressure gauge and fill with air, doing the same for all the tires.
- If you want to check for tread wear, which shows how worn down your tires are, you can use the coin or penny test. Place a penny in the tread with Lincoln's head down and if you can see the top of his head, you will know that the tread is too shallow and the car might be dangerous to drive. Worn-down tires can impact the car's ability to stop and cause blowouts while driving. Your service station may have a digital tread depth gauge that will give you a more precise measurement.

1. **Changing a car tire**

- This may be one of the most useful things you can learn and it isn't as difficult to do as you think. All you need is the right tools and a little bit of knowledge. You should practice a few times at home until you get the knack for it.

- If you get a flat tire while out driving, first check to make sure you have a spare. This is usually in the trunk, under the car upholstery.
- Make sure you have stopped in a safe spot where there is no danger of you being hit by passing traffic. Turn on your hazard lights as a warning to other drivers, and you can also use a warning triangle that should be in the trunk.
- Apply your vehicle's parking brake. You might have wheel wedges to stop it from rolling and if not, look around for a brick or similar-sized stone to use.
- Remove the hubcap or wheel cover with a sharp object, such as a screwdriver, and loosen the lug nuts on the tire with a special wrench. Make sure to loosen them all at the same rate, turning each one in sequence a little bit until they are all loose.
- Place the jack under your vehicle (you should know where to place it depending on your model). You only need to jack it up high enough to be able to remove the flat tire or about six inches off the ground.
- Now you can unscrew the lug nuts completely and remove the tire. Place the spare tire on the car by lining it up with the lug nuts, then tighten each one slowly by hand.
- Lower the car and make sure those lug nuts are tightly screwed on. If anything drops under the car, now is the time to pick it up, and NOT when it is in the air.
- Replace the caps and covers and collect all of your tools. Put them back in the trunk, along with the flat tire.
- You should check the air pressure of the spare tire and go to the nearest gas station or mechanic to have it looked at.

Checking your car fluids

A car runs on 5 main fluids that you will need to keep a regular eye on. There may be others, but these are the ones you can check yourself.

1. **Engine oil**

- This should be checked at least once a month and if you haven't done it before, get someone to help you. Your car's owner or service manual will show where the engine oil dipstick is located. When you have found it, pull it out and wipe it clean with a rag.
- Replace the dipstick and pull it out again. You are checking to see if the engine oil fluid level is in the "safe" zone. If so, no additional oil is needed but if it is low, you need to fill it to the recommended levels.

I. **Coolant**

- You need to check your coolant levels at least every six months, preferably at the beginning of summer and the start of winter. It's the fluid that keeps your car radiator functioning, regardless of the external temperatures.
- First, you need to locate it and it can usually be found inside the radiator but check your car owner's manual to be sure.
- When your car engine is cool, remove the radiator cap and look inside. You will see a line that shows the recommended coolant level. If it is low, you will need to top it up. Then screw the cap back on tightly.

I. **Transmission fluid**

- You should check your car's transmission fluid at least once a month and need to turn your engine on to get an accurate reading.
- Locate the transmission fluid by checking your owner's manual. Here, it's about quality, not quantity, and you are looking at the color of the transmission fluid. It should look red and not smell burned, otherwise, it needs to be replaced. The best way to replace the fluid is to take your car to a mechanic or service center, rather than doing it yourself.

I. **Brake fluid**

- Brake fluid should never be low and can be checked for quality every time your car's oil is changed. You are likely to find the brake fluid reservoir in the engine compartment on the driver's side.
- The fluid should have a golden color and will need replacing if it is brown or looks low. Ask your mechanic or service center to change it for you.

1. **Power steering fluid**

- This is another fluid you should check once a month to see if it is low. The fluid doesn't usually drop suddenly so if you notice that it's well below the right level, take it to your service center for the mechanic to have a look at it.

Changing the air filter

- The air filter in your car helps to keep it free of dirt and dust, which can contaminate your engine system. Ideally, you should change the air filter every 10,000 to 15,000 miles and maybe even more often if you usually drive through dusty or heavily-congested roads.
- You should find the air filter in the car's engine compartment and will need to wipe and remove the top. Remove the oil air filter and wipe clean the housing and filter before replacing it with a new filter.
- After that, replace any screws or clamps and put the top back on. You may prefer to let your mechanic do this, and it's usually included in the yearly car service.

Replace the windshield wiper blades

- This might not seem like a big deal until you get caught in rain and realize your wipers aren't working properly. Streaky windows can obscure your vision and lead to poor road visibility so it's important to make sure your wipers are in tip-top shape.

- To replace the blades, check for the correct blade size. You can buy replacements at most auto parts stores and even at many service stations.
- Remove the old blades, which may need unhooking or snap on and off. Follow the instructions to replace with the new blades.

Jumpstarting a car

Very often, cars won't start because their battery is dead, and if that's the case, you will need someone with another car to help jumpstart it. If you don't feel comfortable doing this or think there may be another problem with your car, call your breakdown service and wait for them to check things out for you. Otherwise, here's what you need to do if you want to jumpstart it:

1. Get out your jumper cables. They should be in the trunk.
2. Find someone with another car that can help you. Their car should have a similar battery voltage to yours.
3. Position the cars face to face but make sure they aren't touching each other.
4. Open the hoods and turn off the engines. Engage the parking brake for extra safety.
5. Each battery should have a positive and a negative terminal, denoted by a + or - sign. They might say POS or NEG and usually have a corresponding red and black color.
6. Attach one red clip of the jumper cables to the positive side of your car's battery.
7. Attach the other red clip to the positive side of the other car's battery.
8. Attach one black clip to the negative side of the other car's battery.
9. Attach the other black clip to an unpainted metal surface away from the battery.
10. Start up the working (donor) vehicle. Let the engine run for a few minutes to charge the battery on your car.
11. Try starting your car and if it works, you can disconnect the

jumper cables. Start with the black (negative cables) first and don't let any of the cables touch while they are still in use.

12. Keep your vehicle running to allow the battery to recharge, which will take at least 15 minutes.

Get to know your car as much as possible, because it will tell you when it needs attention. Keep an eye on the gauges on the dashboard and learn to understand the significance of each one. Take note of the normal sounds your car makes and how it performs when driving so you can spot anything unusual or irregular. When in doubt, always ask a professional, who will check your car for any issues.

Service

Remember that your car should have a full service every year, or after every 10-12,000 miles. The mechanic will usually check for the following, depending on the make and model of your car:

- An engine oil change and/or filter replacement
- Checking lights, tires, exhaust, and operation of brakes and steering
- Ensuring your engine is 'tuned' to run in its peak condition
- Checking hydraulic fluid and coolant levels
- Checking the cooling system (from radiators in your car to pumps and hoses)
- Suspension checks
- Steering alignment
- Testing the car's battery condition

Things you need to keep in your car

You should never drive around without carrying some important tools and accessories in your trunk. These could be crucial if you break down or find yourself in an emergency and knowing how to use them is equally important:

- Jumper cables
- Spare tire

- Air pressure gauge
- Penny (for tread wear test) or tread gauge
- Torque wrench
- Jack stand
- Flares or reflective devices in case you breakdown
- A flashlight
- A car tool kit
- A first-aid kit
- An empty fuel container
- A small shovel for snow
- An ice scraper/brush
- A travel blanket

When driving about, you should always carry with you the right documentation. You can get into real trouble if stopped by a routine traffic stop or are involved in an accident with another driver. Be sure to carry the following with you at all times, even if you are just running to the local grocery store:

1. Driver's License (Essential)
2. Proof of Registration (Essential)
3. Vehicle Insurance (Essential)
4. Vehicle Manual
5. A Pen and Paper
6. Proof of MOT (UK) or Vehicle Inspection Certificate (USA)
7. Emissions Diagnostic Certificate (if applicable)

That's all you need to know about car maintenance for now. Remember that your car needs plenty of love if you want it to run smoothly and take care of you. Treat it with respect, look after it, and always follow the highway code. I don't need to tell you that you should NEVER drink and drive, or use harmful substances that can seriously impair your driving abilities. Both are illegal and extremely dangerous.

Have fun driving your car, safe in the knowledge that you have got everything under control.

Enjoy the ride!

Top tips:

- *Having your own car comes with both independence and responsibility.*
- *Familiarize yourself with the owner's manual as much as you can.*
- *Keeping your car clean inside and out is a great habit to adopt.*
- *Learning how to change a flat tire and jumpstart your car are 2 extremely useful skills.*
- *Checking for the 5 main fluids that keep your car healthy is easy to do.*
- *Remember to take your car for service every 12 months, or 10,000 miles (UK) or after every 12,000 miles (USA).*
- *Always carry the essential tools and accessories with you, as well as all legal documentation.*

7
HOW TO DEAL WITH A ROLLERCOASTER OF EMOTIONS

I have to admit it. I hated being a teenager. It felt like I was on a never-ending rollercoaster of emotional ups and downs that no one understood.

One day I was feeling moody and grumpy, and the next, anxious and stressed, not to mention spotty.

My parents didn't seem to know how to help me and my best friend was also going through her own issues, so it was quite a miserable time in my life. I'm so glad it's all over and done with!

Unfortunately, I didn't have the support I needed to get through those stormy teenage years and I wish I had had someone back then to support me because it was such a difficult 3 or 4 years. If you are around 14, 15, or 16 and struggling with the same issues, I truly feel for you. Trust me when I say that I know exactly what you are going through.

No one ever tells you that adolescence will be so confusing and, even if you are close to your mom or dad, I'm sure you often feel that they really can't help you. You might even unconsciously push them away when they try to help or give you advice because it all seems so cringey.

Not everyone feels that comfortable opening up and talking about their feelings, especially to their parents. It's as if you are in a kind of limbo, no longer a child and not sure what adulthood means. All you know is that life sucks and you can't do anything about it.

With the amount of hormones pumping through your system, it's not surprising that you feel this way. On top of that, all kinds of weird things are going on with your body and it can be overwhelming sometimes. Growing boobs or sprouting facial hair is normal, but it may not feel like that to you. Your friends are all probably going through the same kind of teen terror, so they aren't much help, either.

You might often feel weepy, angry, frustrated, lonely, and go through uncontrollable temper tantrums. One day you're up and the next, flat on your face again. School or college could feel like extra pressure that you can't keep up with and you may lose interest in hobbies that you used to enjoy doing. You most likely suffer from a lot of anxiety and feel like you are in this alone, not knowing who to turn to or what to do.

It may not make much sense when I say this now, but everything you are going through is completely normal. You can learn how to cope with the highs and lows during this difficult transitional period and you'll find help on how to do that in this chapter.

Start off by not being too hard on yourself: everything you are feeling will eventually pass with time and until then, you should be making the most of these teenage years.

What's up with you?

We all feel emotions, no matter what age we are. What happens during adolescence is that you start to experience them very intensely, all at once, and don't have the skills to cope with them. Your brain is still trying to catch up with how to control and express emotions in a way that works for you and those around you and until it does, your moods can be unpredictable.

As you are developing and growing, this can make you more conscious of how you look and harm your self-esteem, especially if you keep comparing yourself to others. When your mates are starting to fill out with muscles and you are still a skinny wimp, this does nothing for your self-image. If, unlike you, your girlfriends have started having their periods, feeling like a late developer may play on your mind in a negative way.

"What's wrong with me?" you may ask yourself and, usually, the answer is, "Nothing!" Everyone grows into adulthood at a different rate, although we know that it begins around the ages of 10-11 years for girls and around 11-12 years for boys.

What's going on?

As you begin to transform into a teenager from a child, certain changes in your brain are going on. Sex hormones start being released from the gonads, which are the ovaries and testes. There's no way of knowing exactly when you will start this process and it can take from 18 months to 5 years. Anything within this range is totally normal, so no need to worry.

These changes are most noticeable in your body, and usually present themselves in the following ways:

Hey Girl!

Around 10-11 years

Your breasts can start growing, and not always at the same rate. One may seem slightly larger than the other and they will feel tender as they develop. Before you start thinking about wearing a bra, which can feel very constricting, a cropped top or sports bra can be much more comfortable.

You have a growth spurt. Your legs may grow more quickly than your torso, making you look out of proportion for a while. During that awkward phase, you might feel clumsy and keep bumping into things - all perfectly normal. The average growth rate for girls is about 5-20 cm until you reach the age of around 16-17 years.

Your body shape will change as your hips widen and you develop a waist.

Your external genitals (vulva) will be more pronounced and you will start to grow hair in that region, which will darken and thicken over time.

Around 12-14 years

You may notice hair growth under your arms.

You will have a clear or white discharge from the vagina several months before your periods start. If it bothers you, you can use slim panty liners but if it feels itchy or painful, it's a good idea to visit your family doctor with an adult.

Your periods will usually start within 2 years of your breast growth, but they may take as long as 4 years.

Oh Boy!

Around 11-12 years

Your external genitals (penis, testes, and scrotum) will start to grow. One testis may appear to be growing faster than the other, which is nothing to worry about. Most men's testes are slightly irregular in size.

You will notice hair growing in your groin area, which will get thicker and darker over time.

Around 12-14 years

You will probably have a growth spurt, with your chest and shoulders broadening. On average, boys grow 10-30 cm until they are around 18-20 years.

You might even notice that your breasts are growing and this will usually go away by itself. If you are worried though, a trip to your family doctor will reassure you.

Around 13-15 years

You will notice more hair growing on your body - under your arms, on the face, chest, and legs, which will thicken over time.

Your brain starts to produce testosterone, the hormone that stimulates the production of sperm in your testes.

You are probably going to experience erections and release sperm (ejaculation), even when you are asleep (wet dreams). This is all perfectly normal and doesn't make you a weirdo.

Around 14-15 years

Your larynx ('Adam's apple' or voice box) will become more prominent as it gets larger and your voice will 'break' and eventually become deeper.

The hormones being released in your body are also responsible for a lot of other physical changes that you have to deal with, regardless of gender.

Growth spurts can make you feel clumsy as your center of gravity changes. This can affect your balance and you might be more accident-prone. It's hard to avoid but you can slow down a bit and take more care of what activities you do, such as climbing or running.

Your muscles may start to grow, (great for the guys) and even your hand-eye coordination will improve, as well as your motor skills, which is a bonus if you like playing sports.

You will also see some weight gain but shouldn't cut down on eating high energy, high protein meals - your body needs these more than ever before. Many teenagers worry about gaining excess weight so it's good to know that your body has its own unique shape. Going on fad diets or binging can lead to serious health problems so if you are worried about your weight, please speak to your parents and get the help of a health professional.

Your sleeping patterns could be disturbed and you may have a tendency to want to stay awake longer at night and sleep in until later the next day. This is a problem if you need to wake up early for school, so it's important to try to maintain a regular sleep schedule and not go to bed too late.

You will notice that you sweat a lot more, especially under your arms, and we talked in the last chapter about the importance of keeping these areas clean. The same goes for your skin and hair, which will be extra oily and often lead to pimples and acne on your face, chest, or back.

While these physical changes are going on in your body, you might feel uncomfortable or embarrassed about them and be over-sensitive to comments about your physical appearance.

Would it help if I told you that every single adult person on this planet has gone through the same thing? It's part of growing up and the survival of our species depends on it so don't give yourself a hard time - you are not alone!

NOTE: If you are concerned about any aspect of your body and the changes going on, speak to a parent or adult you trust. You can even talk to your school counselor and arrange a visit to your family doctor if needs be. Talking about it to friends is fine, but they probably know as little as you do and aren't experts, so could give you the wrong advice.

Brain games

Once you understand that all of these physical changes are healthy and normal, you can begin to think about the mood swings that you are going through. Most of that has to do with your brain, which is growing and developing. By the time you are 6 years old, your brain has already reached about 90-95% of its adult size, but it needs a lot of tweaking until it will begin to function as a normal adult brain. It goes into a kind of hyper mode during teenage years and will keep on until you are in your mid-twenties.

The main change is that it starts to work on the thinking and processing parts, or the 'gray matter'. Some connections within the brain are strengthened while others are fused or done away with altogether, turning it into a more efficient machine. This process includes changes to your prefrontal cortex - the front part of your brain that is responsible for decision-making, planning, problem-solving, and impulse control. It has a lot to do!

While your prefrontal cortex is trying to refine everything, your amygdala steps in to help out. This is a tiny area deep within your brain that has the job of regulating emotions, impulses, aggression, and instinctive behavior. It's not really the amygdala's job to make decisions or solve problems, which explains why everything becomes a bit of a mess.

You can see how that would affect your emotional state, right? In effect, your brain is still under construction and it's a bit like a messy building site inside, full of dangers, risks, and a lot of confusion. Your daily activities contribute, in part, to the final outcome and that's why you really need to think about the way you spend your time. Do you like to do sports, listen to music, learn new languages, or play video games? How do you think these activities are shaping the neural pathways in your brain as you approach adulthood?

Finding your balance

Apart from how you spend your free time, you can focus on ways to deal with all of the emotional turbulence you are experiencing. As I said above, your brain is trying to juggle those decision-making skills with a range of impulses and emotions, so it's tough to find the balance. That's why you are much more prone to mood swings now than when you were younger. By the time you reach adulthood, hopefully, it will all be under control. But for now, what can you do to help yourself?

76

Talking about your feelings is very important, although you might find that difficult to do. Finding the right moment to approach mom or dad may be tricky and they might not have the right approach when it comes to listening. You might find it easier to talk to other people, such as an older sibling or relative, a teacher at school, or a mentor. Sharing your problems with friends is always a great thing to do, even if they don't have all the answers.

If you have a serious problem that you cannot resolve with the people around you, you will find a list of helplines in your area on Google that you can call. Often, it's easier to talk to a stranger than to someone you know, so be sure to reach out if you are feeling overwhelmed or having suicidal thoughts.

Most teenagers, like yourself, will experience these 5 emotions on a regular basis. There are more, but these cover the most common ones:

Depression.

This can feel like short spells of sadness that are triggered by disappointment, discouragement, or a loss. It shouldn't last for long periods of time but if it does (that is, a few weeks or more) and you can't pull yourself out of it, you really need to speak to a medical professional.

Feeling depressed doesn't mean that there is something mentally wrong with you - it's just one of the lows of being a teen and when it appears, you should try to get out and spend more time with friends, go to see a movie, take a walk in the park - anything to change that dark mindset you have fallen into.

Loneliness

This will feel like you are cut-off, disconnected, not understood, and alone. Many teens experience this at some point and with social media probably playing a large part in your life, it's easy to think that everyone else is having a great time while you are alone. The idea that you are missing out on something (FOMO) can make you feel even worse.

Again, spending more time with friends and family is one way to overcome your feelings of isolation. Face-to-face interactions will definitely take your mind off things and the less social media you use, the better. Get off Facebook, Instagram, and Snapchat, and meet your friends in the flesh!

Having a good night's sleep is also a great way to restore your positive energy and exercise will also make you feel less lonely, especially if you take part in team sports or group activities. Try not to sit at home feeling sorry for yourself - it will only make you worse.

Self-rejection

Not liking the person you are becoming or being troubled by your self-image is also something that many teenagers go through. This could be to do with your physical appearance and all of the changes going on in your body. It may also stem from all of the high expectations you feel are being imposed on you at school or in the home, which causes pressure and stress.

Your negative self-image can make you feel that you don't fit in and that you aren't 'good enough, clever enough, handsome enough....' You may fret over your height, weight, what you wear, or even what grades you get. It's important to remember that although things like getting good grades and looking fabulous all the time may seem important, you have to cut yourself some slack. Nobody is perfect and you don't need to aspire to that.

Talk to your parents, teachers, or coach about the high expectations they may have of you and explain how it is making you lose confidence in yourself and creating stress. Stop focusing so much on how you or others look and spend your free time doing the things you enjoy. Your self-esteem will thank you for it.

Anxiety

Anxiety could be described as when you feel acutely worried about something and don't think you can cope with the challenges in life. The idea of having to speak in front of the class, go on a date, or take an exam, can give you palpitations, excessive sweating, and a sense of unease. These are all normal reactions to stress, and most people get anxious about similar things.

It's OK to feel anxious now and again, but it will help to talk to someone about it too. Getting whatever it is off your chest can be so liberating. You also need to practice positive self-talk, saying things like, "I can handle this," "I've got this." Telling yourself you can manage will help to reduce your anxiety and hey, you can always ask someone to help you with a difficult task or project when it all feels like too much to do alone.

Aggression

You might come across as aggressive or even be physically violent. This is like an attempt on your part to take control, or it could be you lashing out because you can't express your feelings in another way. Aggressive behavior usually comes with anger and makes you want to hit out at anything or anyone. You might get away with a certain amount of back-answering your parents or teachers, but being physically violent can seriously harm someone and even lead to criminal prosecution.

When you feel anger welling up inside of you and don't know how to deal with it, it's a good idea to find someone who you can talk to. Your parents and friends may not appreciate your aggressive outbursts so apologize to them and explain that you are finding it difficult to deal with some things at the moment. Hopefully, they will give you the support you need to work things through.

Also, you can try to stop what you are doing, take a deep breath, and think about your behavior. Is it rational, reasonable, fair, and productive, or dangerous, mean, cruel, and harmful? I'm sure that when you catch yourself in this mood, you will see that there are better ways to channel your frustration and anger.

Doing regular exercise can rid you of all that pent-up frustration and give you a chance to 'cool off'. Spend as much downtime as you can, too, hanging out with real friends rather than trying to kill someone on your favorite pc game. If you do feel that you want to lash out at someone, take a break, get some fresh air, listen to chillout music, and allow yourself to calm down.

Like I say, all of these mood swings are normal for most teenagers and part of growing up. You won't always feel this way and you can help yourself by accepting first and foremost that it's all part of the process. It doesn't excuse you from getting involved in criminal activity, indulging in substance abuse, or harming others and if you feel like you have any of those tendencies or urges, find someone to talk to about it.

Peer pressure

The older you get, the more important friends become to you and often, you will feel pressured to go along with them even if you don't want to. This is because you have a need to fit in and that's totally understandable. Being accepted is important to you and peer pressure can be both a positive and negative thing, depending on what you feel compelled to do.

If all of your friends are smoking cigarettes, you might think it's cool to do the same, even though you know how bad it is for your health. That's just one example of the type of behavior you might feel the need to follow so that you can remain popular and wanted by your friends. Other examples could be:

- Wearing the same clothes or having the same funky hairstyle
- Listening to the same music or watching the same TV shows
- Changing the way you talk or the words you use
- Taking risks or breaking rules
- Working less at school
- Taking part in sexual activities
- Smoking, drinking alcohol, or using drugs

Some of the above are harmless and simply help you to create stronger bonds with your friends. The problems arise when you are agreeing to do stuff that isn't your thing and makes you feel uncomfortable, such as taking drugs. As you are growing and developing your own identity, that can often conflict with what your friends are saying or doing, and it can be a very confusing time.

Peer pressure is probably one of the strongest forces you will feel and can even make you go against everything you have been brought up to believe in until now. Learning to know where to draw the line is hard, but you can achieve that by going back to basics.

No matter what your friends are up to, if you don't like it, don't do it. I know that having friends is important to you at this stage of your life, but having the RIGHT friends is even more important. Here are some ways to find the right balance:

Build up your self-confidence by excelling at one thing, be that school-work or a hobby/sport/activity that you like. Confident people don't rely on others to make them feel good about themselves and avoid situations that aren't right for them.

Look at your role models and see how they handle challenges. What would your coach, dad, or mentor do in this situation? How would your mom, aunt, or older sister handle a similar problem?

Be good to yourself, just in the same way you would be kind and compassionate to a sibling or friend. You are still learning and there's no need to beat yourself up for doing something just to fit in. It's a learning process and everyone makes mistakes.

Spend more time with people you admire and talk to them about your issues if you feel able to. You will be surprised at how much you can learn from listening to others and their experiences.

Take up new hobbies or activities where you can make new friends and will have something in common with them. That could be joining a cheerleading team or a Dungeons & Dragons group - whatever it is - you will make friends there for all the right reasons.

Practice saying no when you are asked to go along with suggestions by your friends that you don't feel comfortable with. If they ask you to smoke, simply say no because you don't like the smell of it. If you are a girl and feel pressurized by a boy to engage in sex or other sexual activity with him, say that you are not ready and prefer not to. Be firm when you say no, and make it clear you aren't going to change your mind.

Whenever you find yourself in an unsafe or risky situation, contact an adult immediately and let them know where you are. It's much better to lose face than to put yourself in danger and you should always let a responsible adult know where you are and who you are with, just in case.

Give yourself plenty of options when it comes to making friends. You don't need to try to impress anyone and a true friend will value you for who you are, not for who they want you to be.

I hope you've learned a lot more about yourself in this chapter and found some ways to get through these teenage years with fewer tears and tantrums.

Next, we are going to be looking at ways to have a positive body image and how to be more resilient when the going gets tough.

See you soon!

Top tips:

- *Being a teenager is a rough ride, but everyone has gone through it.*
- *All the mood swings you experience are a natural part of growing up.*
- *Girls' bodies go through different changes to boys and it can take a while before you feel comfortable in your own skin.*
- *The brain is trying to find its balance and this can cause havoc with your emotions.*
- *You can overcome intense feelings of loneliness, depression, self-rejection, anxiety, and aggression.*
- *Peer pressure will test your ability to be led astray but you can resist it.*

❦ 8 ❦

STAYING POSITIVE WHEN
TIMES GET TOUGH

D on't you just hate it when adults say things like, "Cheer up, things aren't that bad...?"

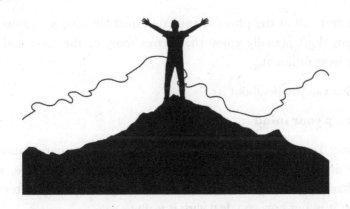

It's so annoying - especially when they know nothing about what you are going through. You might have a hundred exams coming up at school, have just been dumped by your latest girlfriend/boyfriend, or are feeling crushed because you didn't make it onto the athletics team. And they say, "Cheer up?" Grrrrr!

Every day may seem like a battle, starting with getting out of bed. When that alarm goes off, all you really want to do is roll over and go back to dreamland. But your mom is banging on your door, telling you that you are going to be late. You have to sprint to the bus stop, don't have time for breakfast, realize you have forgotten your math book at home, and a massive zit has just erupted on your chin. How much worse can your day get?

Weekends aren't much better. Your dad has just told you that you are grounded for answering back (yeah, right), you have tons of boring homework to do, your best friend isn't responding to your texts, and you feel kind of miserable. What's to look forward to but more of the same? Your life is an endless cycle of home, school, nagging, disappointments, AND your wifi sucks!

I get it. All of these things can wear you down when all you want to do is chill out with your friends and have some fun. It's your life, but you don't have the means yet to enjoy that full independence, so you just have to suck it up. It's no wonder that so many teenagers suffer from anxiety, mood swings, and frustration.

Apart from all of the physical and emotional challenges, the majority of teens don't actually enjoy themselves most of the time and wish things were different.

So, what can you do about it?

Make up your mind

The way I see it, you have two choices. You can either continue to complain and vent about all the bad things going on in your life, or you can change your mindset and start to see things differently. After all, it is what it is, but how you deal with it is up to you.

Believe me when I say that most people go through difficult times in their lives, and it doesn't get any easier as you reach adulthood. There will ALWAYS be those external pressures, whether that's with your job or career goals, within your family, with friends, and the world in general.

It's not as if everything suddenly falls into place and you never have to face difficult decisions or circumstances. Even having a lot of money isn't going to free you of personal problems, no matter how much of it you have.

If you continue to moan and feel wretched, you won't be doing yourself any favors. Sure, it's hard to be optimistic when you feel like you are in a dark tunnel with no light at the end. Time seems to drag when you are in your teens and it's not easy to convince yourself that this period of your life will ever be over.

On the other hand, if you can try to change your perspective on things, I can assure you that you will stop focusing on the bad and feel a lot more positive about everything. Are you ready and willing to at least give it a go? If your answer is yes, read on.

This chapter is all about feeling good within yourself and when you can achieve that, you'll see life through a totally different lens. Like I say, adulthood also has its challenges, and the sooner you learn to build up your self-confidence and greater mental resilience, the better for you.

You could think of it as every cloud having a silver lining, which is the way optimists view life. They know that the black clouds are there, but also know that when the storm passes, the sun is going to shine. It's something you can't deny, but you have probably been focusing on those storm clouds instead of seeing beyond them.

I don't want to bore you with lots of scientific stats and data, but all of the research clearly shows that the ability to see that silver lining and remaining optimistic goes hand in hand with positive emotional well-being, better health, lower levels of depression, and even a longer life. What's not to love about that!

You might be wondering how that's possible. Well, we've known for a long time that stress negatively affects our mental and physical health. In the same way, seeing the bright side of life reduces stress and helps us to cope better with problems, unpredictable emotions, and offers us a healthier lifestyle.

The best place to start changing how you deal with all of the challenges is within yourself. I'm sure that a lot of your misery boils down to your low self-esteem. This is when you don't believe you are capable of improving your life because you are not good enough, strong enough, smart enough, pretty enough, and so on.

Because you lack that self-confidence, you can end up feeling powerless and it's this sense of hopelessness that often leads to anxiety and the inability to handle pressure. It definitely stops you from believing that things will get better in the future and keeps you in a constant state of misery. You feel unlovable, incompetent, unworthy, unable, and all of these negative self-doubts can be overwhelming at your age.

Here's the thing: the majority of high school students are going through exactly the same thing as you. Their problems might be slightly different from yours but the one thing you all have in common is a lack of self-esteem and confidence. The kind of things that many teens worry about include:

- Being overweight
- Not feeling attractive enough
- Not having enough muscles (usually boys)
- Being bullied/trolled
- Body shaming
- Negative self-image
- Peer pressure and wanting to fit in
- Not being good enough or not measuring up
- Not having enough friends/not being popular

All of the above are legitimate concerns, especially when you are at an age where your body is changing and your emotions can be up and down from one day to the next. The best way to deal with these worries is to strengthen your sense of self and be proud of who you are, no matter what.

Let's look at some ways of doing exactly that.

1. **Silence that inner critic**

86

Your impression of yourself is created largely by your thoughts. It's you who feels too fat, too thin, too slow, too dumb, too useless. Even if someone else has told you any of these things, you are the one who has taken it to be true. We are our own worst enemies in many ways, often generating negative self-talk which only makes us feel worse about ourselves.

Just in the same way that you drown out what's going on around you by listening to music, you can silence the voice in your head that is talking down to you all the time. You don't need to listen to it and shouldn't let it take away your power. You are an amazing person, even if you have flaws, but that voice feeds on your doubts and insecurities. The next time you catch yourself thinking, "I'm so fat" or "I'm not smart enough," speak up for yourself and change the narrative.

Repeat to yourself, "My bodyweight doesn't define me" or "I am capable of doing whatever I put my mind to" and keep doing so until you have silenced the inner critic and found a new, more positive voice.

1. Stop comparing yourself to others

I know how important it is to fit in with your friends and be the same as them. You want to be just as attractive, sporty, cool, or popular, and often don't feel that way.

You might focus on your imperfections, obsess over your weight or physical shape, and worry that others don't like you so much. On top of that, you are bombarded with images of perfection on social media every day and see fabulous influencers leading fantastic lives.

Having a positive body image is very important as it gives you the confidence you need to go through life with your head held high. Succumbing to the pressure to change the way you look just so you fit in can be demoralizing and exhausting, as well as do little for your self-esteem.

I think you are smart enough to know that we can't believe everything we see on the internet and that social media is NOT real life. Nobody is living that perfect dream and even if they are, what difference should it make to you? You will NEVER be exactly the same as somebody else because you are unique. It's just not possible to have the same hair as your best friend or the same personality, and thank goodness for that.

When you begin to appreciate your individuality, you won't feel the need to compare yourself with others anymore. You can begin by looking at yourself in the mirror and repeating five times, "I am beautiful/I am handsome/I am a great person/I am unique." Do this once or twice a day until you start believing it because it's the only truth you need.

1. Find your strengths and weaknesses

We all have good and bad points, and getting to identify them can be very empowering. It helps us to learn where our boundaries lie and what resources we can count on to overcome challenges. It's an easy exercise to do, and all you need is a pen or paper, or make a note on your smartphone.

Make two headings - Strengths and Weaknesses. Then spend some time thinking about what you are going to write. It could look something like this:

Strengths

I'm good at art

I'm a generous person

I like helping around the house

I'm a great swimmer

Weaknesses

I'm a little bit lazy

I don't like expressing myself

I'm very shy

I'm no good at math

Once you have made your own list, focus on those strengths and give yourself a pat on the back. You should feel proud of yourself for having them. As for your weaknesses, consider how important they are in your life.

What would you like to change or improve on? If, for example, you are shy, think about how that is impacting your ability to make friends. Is there anything you can do to overcome it, such as finding the courage to join a new club or group? For some people, being shy isn't a big deal, so it's also a great chance for you to consider why you think being shy is a weakness in the first place.

Be sure to look at your list often and add to it or delete certain things as time goes by. I never felt like I was good at math when I was at school, and failed all of my exams miserably. I truly believed that I was completely useless at the subject and it wasn't until I went to college and had to do Statistics as one of the modules that I realized something. It wasn't that I was bad at math after all. I had simply talked myself into believing it and had given up trying long ago. When I started studying Statistics, which has a lot of math, I found it easy because I was more motivated to succeed.

1. **Forget 'What if'**

I know the feeling - your mind is racing with all of the things that could go wrong. Whether you've got a romantic first date planned, an important football game, or a school trip, you are constantly worried about it being a total flop.

It's OK to be worried when you want everything to go well, but you can't control the future. Whatever goes wrong is usually unpreventable so what's the use in painting a picture of doom and gloom now? It stops you from enjoying the present moment and takes all the pleasure out of looking forward to an upcoming event.

Instead of wondering, 'What if I make a mistake or do something stupid?' focus on how great it is going to be. It makes no sense to expect a catastrophe or worry about how you will handle things. Trust in yourself and your abilities and go on that date full of confidence, play that game to win. Whatever the outcome, you can say that you did your best and enjoyed it at the same time!

1. **Know your triggers**

We are all triggered by different things, which set off a variety of emotions. It's important to know what your triggers are, so you can avoid them or learn how to deal with them. For example, if you suffer from low self-esteem, spending an hour on Instagram looking at picture-perfect men or women is going to trigger even more self-loathing.

If you feel hopeless and pessimistic in general, watching the news may cause you to feel even worse, so it's better to watch something more upbeat instead.

We can't always avoid the people around us and, very often, they can trigger feelings of anger, embarrassment, frustration, or worthlessness. What you can do is take control of how you process those emotions. As soon as you feel anger welling up inside you after something someone has said about you, stop to think about how much power you are giving them. Is it really in your best interests to let someone else dictate your emotions?

You need to work at this because, as you grow older, these triggers can become long-term habits that are hard to break. The way you react to others says more about how you feel about yourself than it does about them. Don't let others decide how you are going to feel or how to live your life. It's not up to them.

1. **Practice healthy habits**

The harder you are on yourself, the more difficult you will find it to have a positive mindset. Not only that, but you are much more likely to experience unpleasant sensations such as fatigue, headaches, or the feeling of being run down. A lot of teens have very disturbed sleep patterns or suffer from sleep deprivation. They don't always eat right and, on top of that, experience a lot of stress, which can wreak havoc on the immune system.

You can help yourself to deal with life's ups and downs a lot better if you establish some basic healthy habits. These could be:

- Going to bed each night at a set time
- Not scrolling through your newsfeed before going to sleep
- Eating breakfast, even if it's just a slice of toast
- Making sure you eat a healthy lunch and dinner
- Replacing sugary and fatty snacks with fresh fruit or high-protein snacks
- Showering regularly and wearing clean clothes
- Taking care of your appearance
- Setting a daily schedule for tasks you need to do
- Planning something enjoyable for the weekend, preferably with friends

These are all very easy suggestions to apply and will have a positive effect on your overall well-being. A good night's sleep, a healthy diet, being organized, and having fun will do wonders for your confidence and enable you to take on any challenge.

1. **Start your day with positivity**

This may sound like one of those icky feel-good quotes, but every day really is a new day. It's a chance for you to begin anew, with more positivity than you had yesterday. I bet you are wondering what difference that will make. Actually, it will make all the difference.

Instead of carrying over with you from the day before all the stresses, pressures, and negative thoughts, you have the opportunity to begin with a clean slate and that's a great way to start your day. Think of it as an update to your laptop or phone - the hardware is the same but the new updates make everything run so much smoother, without the lag.

1. **Think positively**

It's not easy to be optimistic all the time but it is a skill you can teach yourself. For example, instead of seeing the worst in any given scenario, look for the good in it. This is one way to reprogram your brain to see the brighter side of life, even when things go wrong. When you wake up tomorrow morning, instead of saying, "Oh, it's Monday again and that sucks," make a positive statement like, "Yeah! Monday is here and it's a brand new week!" It won't change what goes on in your week, but it will help you to sail through it will less negativity and stress.

1. **Focus on others**

By helping others, you can raise your feel-good levels and who wouldn't want that? There's a lot to be said for giving to other people instead of dwelling on your own problems. Often, you will find that your problems are not nearly half as important. They may turn out not to be problems at all. A little compassion and loving kindness can go a very long way so think about what you can do to help someone out each day.

You will gain a lot of perspective on what is important in life and it can be a very humbling experience. They say that charity begins at home, so you could offer to help out more around the house, help a younger sibling with their homework, or take the dog for a walk more often. You can volunteer some of your free time to help out at an animal shelter, local children's hospital, or visit an elderly neighbor who might enjoy the company.

Whenever you help others, you are helping yourself to grow into a person with integrity and self-respect. This will shape your character and arm you with the strength to deal with life's challenges both now and in the future.

1. **Give thanks**

One of the things you will gain from helping others is a wider perspective on how fortunate you are. While you are complaining about not having the latest iPhone or Nike sneakers, many people are doing without basic things like companionship or a roof over their heads.

You don't have to feel guilty about this, which isn't a productive emotion, but it can inspire you to appreciate what you do have in your life.

Feeling gratitude will fill you with renewed energy and positivity even when things aren't going your way. If you can think about all the positive aspects of your life and fully appreciate them, you will be able to manage hardships much better. Not having that latest iPhone won't seem so bad after all and you don't need to feel miserable about it anymore! Express gratitude before you go to sleep every night, just by saying, "Thank you," and you will sleep a lot better.

1. Knowing what you can and cannot change

There's a knack to knowing what you can or can't change and learning to accept that. If, for example, you have ever had to stay at home because you were sick, you will know how frustrating that was. Not being able to get out, see your friends, attend concerts or sporting events can be hard at your age.

The reality is that when you accept the way things are, you can make the most of your time at home and will be much less likely to feel frustrated or moody. Acceptance of what we cannot change comes with wisdom and it's not an easy thing to access, but it can be done. When you acknowledge what you can or can't control, it is possible to have some peace of mind. This is extremely useful as you travel through life because it removes a lot of the stress that comes with trying to swim against the current. Knowing when to take action and when to let go is power!

1. Having things to look forward to.

Even if you don't feel like life is sweet now, it will improve. As time goes by, we are all moving from one phase of our lives to the next and your teenage years won't last forever. If you are really having a hard time, it's a good idea to set yourself small treats - things to look forward to in the near future - instead of wishing your life away as you wait for adulthood to arrive.

You don't need to focus on things that are expensive or difficult to achieve. It's more about anything that makes you happy, whether that's going ice-skating at the weekend or attending a rock concert next month. When you have something to look forward to, life doesn't feel half as bad.

I. **Learning from your mistakes**

In this learning game of life, we often trip up, make mistakes, fail, and have regrets. You might still be feeling annoyed about the time you missed that easy shot in volleyball or failed your driving test. We all win some and lose some, and that's just the way it is, but knowing how to learn from our mistakes and move on is priceless.

Obviously, when you feel like a failure, it can seriously affect your confidence levels. You might hate yourself for being such a loser and be so traumatized that you never want to try for anything again. You could have done something that had serious repercussions, such as crashing your new car, or getting into trouble with your parents because you stayed out too late. There are plenty of things that can go wrong, and they often do.

Having said that, rather than being dragged down by your mistakes, it's much better to see them as life lessons. What can you learn from them? What would you do if you found yourself in that situation again? These are the questions you can ask yourself and when you spend some time thinking about them, you will be better prepared for the future. You can forget what went wrong in the past and focus on how to make things go right the next time around.

Finally, have some pizza

With all of the pressures on you and the mixed-up emotions you are experiencing as a teenager, it's easy to feel totally overwhelmed and misunderstood. That's why having a clear image of your own self-worth is really important and you can start to nurture this by drawing a circle. Imagine a pie diagram, or in this case, a pizza, with each segment representing one aspect of who you are. The size of each of your wedges shows how important you think each aspect is.

94

For example, my pizza might be cut into 4 equally large pieces: each piece symbolizes the 4 main aspects of my self-worth. I could say 1 is my performance at work, 2 is my health, 3 is my appearance, and 4 is my creativity. All of these are equally important to me, so I want to spend an equal amount of time on each one in order to feel content and fulfilled.

What about you?

What would your pizza look like? How many slices would it have?

Would your slices include spending time with friends, studying, family, music, sport, hiking... anything else?

When you've made your pizza, not only will it help you to stay focused on whatever is important to you but it can reveal where you need to pay more attention. Your self-worth lies in knowing who you are, and this activity can help you to stay true to your values, whatever problems arise.

There is always a silver lining, but you need to look for it. It's not easy to be optimistic when you feel really down, but the only way is up if you want to enjoy life.

Find the good in the bad, see the light in the darkness, and trust in yourself - you can do this!

Top tips:

- *Having a positive mindset will help you to enjoy your life much more.*
- *Don't believe your inner critic - it's usually lying.*
- *You are unique and don't need to compare yourself with other people.*
- *Identifying your strengths and weaknesses is a useful tool.*
- *Focus on the future with optimism and forget 'end of the world' scenarios.*
- *Healthy habits bring peace of mind.*
- *Giving to others and expressing gratitude are very empowering.*
- *Your past failures are the key to your future successes.*
- *Always look for the silver lining.*

❦ 9 ❦

GET SOCIAL & MAKE MORE
FRIENDS

How many times have you heard your folks say, "When we were young, we didn't have any of this technology. We used to go out and spend time with friends?" Cringe moment!

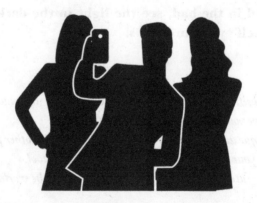

If your parents are old enough to be Generation Xs or even Boomers, they obviously don't know what they are talking about. Technology is great and the digital age is here to stay. They have no idea that you talk to your friends much more now than they would have when they were younger. In fact, you hang out with them online all day, chatting, playing games, watching Netflix together, without even needing to be in the same room.

I think that if your parents do hark on about the 'good old days' before smartphones or laptops, it's because they are worried that you don't have any REAL interaction with friends or not as much as they think you should. They probably feel that you spend far too much time in your room on your PC or phone and would prefer to see you getting out more.

There's also a lot of coverage in the media about teens spending too much time online, getting addicted to video gaming, as well as the risk of online grooming and cyberbullying. That can cause parents to worry a lot, especially if they don't know what you are doing in your room.

No doubt, you know what I'm talking about but you can't just go offline and lose that connection with your friends. You've grown up in the digital culture and it's a part of your life. You probably have a lot of friends on social media platforms like Facebook, Instagram, and TikTok and don't see any problem.

A word about social media

There are a lot of good reasons why you love social media – you can create your own identity, build social networks, get support when using them, and find people with the same interests as you. It's a place where you can express yourself freely, learn lots of cool stuff, and interact across borders at the swipe of a screen. It stops you from feeling so lonely in many ways and it's a lot of fun.

But there is a downside to overuse, especially if you spend so much time logged in that you are losing sleep, or succumbing to peer pressure to do certain things. Some researchers say that the more time you spend on social media as a teen, the more risk there is of you suffering from poor mental health and a lower level of well-being.

That could be to do with how emotionally invested you get during your time there. You might receive negative comments on posts that you take to heart, see others living a 'great life' while you have problems at home, and these kinds of things can raise your anxiety levels.

Feeling dissatisfied with your own life or the way you look in comparison to images you see on social media might eventually affect your self-esteem and confidence, which is the last thing you need. It can also make you feel even more lonely, even though the purpose of it all is to 'connect'. A lot of parents are concerned about the impact of their teens spending too much time on social media, and you can understand why, even if you don't agree with them.

While I totally get how cool these platforms are, there is much more to life. Nothing can be a substitute for real interaction, meeting people face to face, and sharing time together in the real world. But that can take you out of your comfort zone, making you feel awkward and not sure of yourself.

It's one thing to exchange messages with the boy you like from school on Viber or WhatsApp, and quite another to actually have a conversation with him when he's standing right next to you. Chatting to strangers online is easier as well, and making new friends there is much less stressful than trying to hit it off with someone you hardly get the chance to talk to at school.

What are social skills and why do you need them?

Believe it or not, there will be times in your life when you will need to have a face-to-face conversation, communicate your thoughts and feelings verbally, create and maintain relationships (in your future job or while at university), make new friends, and handle difficult interactions with others. You need social skills to pull these off, which will help you to navigate life more successfully.

We know from the experts that young people with advanced social skills are four times more likely to graduate, be successful in their career, enjoy greater independence, and are more emotionally balanced. They are also usually better at decision-making and problem-solving, as well as having stronger social connections. You could say that social skills are quite important and if you feel that you could do with improving yours, I'm going to explain how to.

You can divide social skills into four main groups:

1. **Survival skills**: Things like listening and following directions seem like basic skills, but how many of them are you really good at?
2. **Interpersonal skills:** Joining a conversation, taking turns to talk, sharing your thoughts and emotions, are just some of the things that you might have difficulty with.
3. **Problem-solving skills:** These include asking for help, deciding what to do or what action to take in a particular situation. These might be difficult to do, especially if you have been relying on others to make decisions for you up until now.
4. **Conflict resolution skills:** Dealing with differences of opinion, knowing how to be a good loser, and admitting when you are wrong are skills you will definitely need to have as a teenager. It comes with the territory.

How you can improve your social skills

We are going to take a look at some of the ways you can be more socially effective, even if you don't feel confident enough at the moment. You can learn how to improve the way you interact with others and make new friends, and it's not as difficult as it seems.

Survival skills

A lot of the time, you might be living in your own world, earplugs in and music on. That's fine, but knowing how to listen to other people is pretty important, especially if they are giving you instructions or directions. One way to do this is by establishing eye contact. It's a lot easier to follow what someone is saying if you are looking at them.

When mom or dad are telling you about the schedule for the week ahead, turning away means you aren't really paying attention to what they are saying. It can also come across as disrespectful and I'm sure you've been told so a few times in the past. When they say, "Look at me when I'm talking to you," it's probably because they feel you are ignoring them. So, establishing eye contact is an important social skill. You might not even realize that you are doing it, which is why I'm here to remind you.

Try holding eye contact with the person talking to you for at least 50% of the time if you can. You don't need a calculator for that; just use your common sense. Another way to handle it is to hold eye contact for about five to ten seconds if you can before looking away slowly. Paying attention when the other person is talking through eye contact helps you to follow what they are saying and to remember what they said later on. You also avoid coming across as bored or uninterested, which is not something you want to do.

Interpersonal skills

You might greet your friends with a high-five, a 'wassup bro' or a 'hey girl', but that doesn't really work when you need to address a teacher, employer, college professor, or someone in authority. Using someone's name when you interact with them will establish a more positive connection and leave a much better impression. Introduce yourself clearly too and add any other information you think is important, such as where you live, what class you are in, and so on.

After that, knowing how to hold a conversation might be a bit tricky. You have to actually follow a dialogue that doesn't involve emojis or GIFs, and that's not something you are used to doing. One way to crack this skill is by being prepared to ask questions, which takes the heat off you having to talk too much. The more questions you ask the other person, the less you will need to say, which I know probably suits you just fine. When my son was growing up, he reached what I called his 'caveman phase', where he seemed unable to answer anything I asked him with more than a grunt. I kind of understood his reluctance to engage in conversation with me but could see that this wasn't going to go down well if that's how he responded to his teacher or college professor. Are you currently going through that phase?

Here are some examples of how you can respond in an adult conversation:

Adult: *How are you today?*

You: *I'm great, thank you. How are you?*

Adult: *How is school/college going?*

You: *It's all good. What's going on with your job?*

I know this might not sound very realistic, but I think you get my point. Show as much interest as you can in the other person and let them do the talking. They will be pleased that they have your attention!

When you look at someone as they talk to you, you also get a lot of clues about them by their facial expressions and body language. It can even make up around 60% of what they are really feeling or thinking, so take notice of those cues and learn to respond appropriately. Things like crossing their arms may mean they feel defensive while looking flushed could signify they are embarrassed and it's useful to understand whatever they are expressing.

Don't keep looking at your phone when you are talking to someone else: it will seem as if you are uninterested in what they are saying and can be annoying, as well as downright rude. If you want to impress the new girl you just met in the university cafeteria, glancing at your phone all the time while she is talking will not go down well, trust me. Imagine how you would feel if someone did the same to you!

When you show that you understand what the other person is feeling, you gain their trust, which helps to form strong relationships. You can do this by nodding when they are talking to you, and interjecting with phrases such as, "I know what you mean," "Yes, I see..." Expressing empathy is a great way to bond with someone and a skill very much linked to emotional intelligence.

Problem-solving skills

Part of going through adolescence before reaching adulthood involves having to start making decisions of your own. Your parents or other adults can guide you and share their opinions, but sometimes it's a decision you need to make on your own. Deciding what to study at college, which job to apply for, or where to find accommodation are all on you and that might feel quite stressful.

Here's a step-by-step guide to take the pressure off decision-making and finding solutions to problems, whatever they are:

Identify the problem. What exactly is the issue? Who is affected by it? You can write it down so it's clearly explained in black and white. It may be things like which assignment to do next, how to get home safely from a party, or which university to apply to.

Why is it a problem? How important is it to you? Why do you need to resolve it now? What will happen if you don't? When you think about the answers to these questions, it will give you the time to consider each one clearly and find possible outcomes that work for you.

Brainstorm the problem with an adult. This is useful as it might bring things to the table that you hadn't thought about. List any ideas that come up and reflect on them later while thinking about which one seems the best way to move forward.

Look at the pros and cons. Cross off your list any ideas that are unworkable or unrealistic and once you only have a few possible options left, rate them on a scale of 1 to 10, with 1 being not good and 10 being very good.

If you are still undecided, go back to step 3 and look for different options. Sometimes, there is no perfect 10, in which case you have to make a compromise, and that's also a reflection on life itself.

Put your plan into action. Write down the strategy you are going to use and think of how you will go about achieving your goal. What actions do you need to take? Can anyone help you with them? What sort of time frame are you working with?

Assess how well your plan is going. In time, look at how things are working out. If you have met problems on the way, how can they be resolved? Is there anything you need to change? If you feel you have made the wrong decision, go back to step 1 and start over again.

Conflict resolution skills

Life is full of conflicts and you just can't get away from them. You might fight or argue with your parents, siblings, friends, or people you don't even know that well but learning how to come out of them unscathed is important. The way you deal with conflict now will not be appropriate by the time you reach adulthood so learning how to resolve any is vital. It's one thing to kick your kid brother because he borrowed your shower gel and quite another to behave in the same way when a future colleague uses your pen.

Here's an easy guide to work through conflict and, hopefully, come out of it in one piece:

Rule 1: Conflict happens often but isn't necessarily a bad thing. It can be an opportunity to resolve an issue or clear the air, but you have to learn how to deal with it wisely.

Rule 2: Rather than trying to ignore the issue, it's best to get it out in the open. It could be that you have had a big argument with your best friend or feel your parents are always on your back. These kinds of things need to be tackled head-on because they don't usually go away by themselves.

Rule 3: Think of it in terms of the problem, and not the person. Conflict arises from differences in opinions or perspectives, and not because of who you are. It's not that your parents dislike you; they may just dislike your behavior.

Rule 4: Listen carefully to what the other person is saying. Is there any basis in their opinion? Do you think they might have a point?

Rule 5: Stand up for what you believe in but don't come across as aggressive or overbearing. Avoid being a pushover too, because this could end up in you agreeing to things that don't reflect who you really are.

Rule 6: Focus on the issue at hand and don't start dragging up what was said or done in the past. You won't resolve anything in this way.

Rule 7: Sulking or locking yourself in your bedroom isn't the way to sort out any issues. Not talking to your friend will prolong the stalemate and get you nowhere. Talking it out is always the best way to resolve conflict.

Rule 8: Put yourself in the other person's shoes and try to understand where they are coming from. If you want them to show you empathy, you have to be prepared to do the same.

Rule 9: Learn to apologize if you are in the wrong. Admitting that you made a mistake is a sign of strength, not weakness, so be prepared to say sorry when you need to.

You can use all of the above skills to help you make new friends, too. If you don't think you need to do so because you have a lot of school friends you have known for years, that's fine.

On the other hand, you could have just moved to a new school or area and don't know anyone at all. That can be a very lonely experience, especially at your age. Maybe you are preparing to leave home to go to college or university soon and are worried about how you are going to make new friends when the time comes. It's a daunting thought that you might be stressing about now.

You are welcome to read the book I wrote on this very subject, with the title, **How To Make Friends Easily.** You can find it as an ebook or paperback on Amazon, as well as on Audible as an audiobook.

In the book, I talk about all of the ways you can meet new people, strike up friendships, and form close bonds for life. It's definitely worth a read! Many of the tips in the book relate directly to teenagers like yourself, and you will find some of the main ones below.

Get out and about

If you have moved to a new area because of school, college, or for work, where you know no one, making new friends isn't as hard as it sounds. There are thousands of people just like you who are feeling alone and want to strike up new friendships. In class, at your favorite new resto or coffee shop, around the neighborhood, at your local sports club or gym, there are a lot of opportunities to make new friends.

Get out of the house as much as possible and meet up with others who share your interests or passions. Look out for activities going on in your area that you can check out or organize your own social events and invite people to join. The more active you are, the easier it will be to meet new people.

Learn the art of connecting

Trying to find something to say when you meet someone new can be nerve-racking. What if you say something dumb or the other person isn't interested in talking to you?

Remember that it's a good idea to ask the other person questions about themselves and to let them do the talking. As long as you don't appear to be interrogating them, but are genuinely interested in what they have to say, it's all good.

Ask the kind of questions that need more than a yes or no answer, with things like, "What are you enjoying about your university course?" or, "What do you think of the social life here?"

Maintain good eye contact with them and show you are paying attention but respect their personal space - no one likes to feel that being invaded. Offer to exchange profiles or phone numbers if the chat went well and arrange to meet up again.

Be yourself

If you are serious about making good friends, there's no point in pretending to be someone you aren't. It's Ok to be yourself, flaws and all, and genuine connections are always based on honesty. Anyway, people will be able to see through your lies very quickly, so be open, genuine, and willing to trust. It's the best way to make real friends.

Be a good friend

In order to find and keep good friends, you have to be prepared to make the effort. It's almost impossible to establish any kind of meaningful connection if you are always unavailable, don't keep in contact with them, or fail to meet up often. Friendships are built on mutual trust and understanding, which needs time and work. Be there when they need you but be sure to set your boundaries too. Giving everything up in order to keep them happy isn't a balanced friendship and you will soon find that out so start off as you mean to go on, respecting both their boundaries and your own.

Don't stay in a toxic relationship

You should never go along with a friendship if it is harming your self-esteem, or affecting your physical and emotional health. That need to fit in can often be so strong that you might find yourself tempted to do things you will later regret. True friends will NEVER ask you to do anything that isn't good for you or expect you to bend to their will. It can be hard feeling lonely but hanging out with people who aren't good for you can be catastrophic.

Choose your friends based on YOUR needs and preferences and hang out with people who make you feel good about yourself. A true friend is there to support you, not bring you down and this goes for online friends as well.

If you feel that a friend of yours is forcing you into any kind of coercive relationship, seek help from an adult and get sound advice on how to deal with it. It's OK to ask for help, by the way - adults do it all the time!

There's nothing better in life than having close friends with whom you can enjoy spending time. They give you the space you need to be yourself, to have a laugh, to be silly, and to share your problems with.

Having good friends is probably one of the most important thing you can have and many of your current school friends will be here for you for life. You might lose touch with others as the years pass and circumstances change, but remembering all the good times you had with them is something to treasure.

Your teenage years can be confusing times, but with the help of good friends, you'll get through it all. As you go off into the big wide world in a new town or city, you will need to make new friends. This doesn't mean that you forget your old ones, just that you have different needs now, and that's completely normal.

It can be challenging to cope with growing up, but I hope you've found some good ideas in this chapter to help you on your way.

Top tips:

- *Social media is a part of life but not a substitute for real life.*
- *The four main social skills will help you to navigate relationships much easier.*
- *Better communication, being able to resolve conflict, and problem-solving are essential life skills.*
- *Making new friends requires some time and effort but you won't regret it.*

A PERSONAL MESSAGE FROM REBECCA

I t's tough being a teen, both for you and your parents. Neither of you knows how to handle a lot of the baggage that comes with being at that age so it can be a learning process for both.

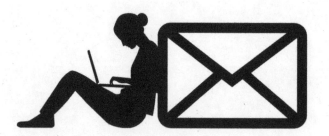

As far as you are concerned, you have to deal with a lot of things you aren't equipped to handle. Nobody told you it would be like this.

You have the internal turmoil of emotions that can bring chaos on a daily basis. Your mood swings seem uncontrollable and will often trigger arguments and conflicts between you and your friends or family. Hormonal changes also lead you to make rash decisions and act on impulse without thinking things through

You have all of the physical changes going on that can make you feel awkward and embarrassed. This can make you struggle with low self-confidence and self-esteem as you measure yourself against others.

You have the external pressures of school, college, house rules, parental expectations, and your peers. This can be overwhelming and lead to a lot of anxiety and stress. Spending time online can seem like an escape from reality but it can have a lot of negative side effects.

You desperately want to fit in and might find yourself in situations that you aren't equipped to handle. Craving attention can lead you down the wrong path and have serious consequences.

You also want your independence, feel suffocated by your parents, and need to find your own identity. Going against the norms can cause even further conflict and the more restricted you feel, the more rebellious you become.

Having brought up two kids of my own, I've gone through those teenage years and know how difficult they can be for everyone. There is no rule book out there for parents on how to help their children get through this phase of their lives so a lot of it is learning as we go. What you need to know is that your parents have your best interests at heart and even if they seem too strict, unreasonable, or heavy-handed, most of the time it's to protect you.

When you neglect your schoolwork, stop showering, drink alcohol, take drugs, or act recklessly, that's a BIG worry for your folks. You might see your behavior as acceptable but you really don't have the life experience or wisdom to understand the consequences of your actions. That's why you need parents to guide you, so how about cutting them some slack?

Sometimes, it can feel like they are against you because they don't care about you and I can see how that plays out. You don't get why they won't let you stay out late and have fun. When they forbid you to get a tattoo or piercing like your friends, it's as if they don't want you to fit in. If they ground you for getting bad grades this semester, it's like they want to see you suffer, right?

Trust me when I tell you that life isn't always easy. We all have to follow rules, behave in a way that's acceptable to society, abide by the law, and get on with others. That doesn't mean that you can't be your own person or live the way you want to live. You can do all of that, in time, but at the moment, you aren't ready. That's what being a teenager is all about: testing boundaries, discovering more about yourself, and learning how to be an adult.

It can be a rough ride, but you will get there in the end.

If you feel that you need to talk to a professional about anything that is worrying you, be sure to reach out to your parents or older relatives, teacher, school counselor, coach, help hotlines, or any other adult you trust. We all need help at times and there's no shame in asking for it.

Struggling alone with your worries isn't usually the best way to sort anything out so no matter how small your problem seems, talk to someone about it who can give you the guidance and support that you need.

In the meantime, enjoy these teenage years as you explore your identity, discover more about yourself, and learn how to ease into adulthood without causing too much damage!

Have fun because your wonderful life is just getting started!

Make An Author Happy Today!

I hope you found this book helpful. If you did, I would be eternally grateful if you could spend a couple of minutes writing a review on Amazon - or Audible if you bought the Audiobook.

When you post a review, it makes a huge difference in helping more readers find my book.

Your review would make my day

Thanking you in advance

Rebecca

Other books by me:

How To Make Friends Easily

Love Yourself Deeply

The Art Of Manifesting Money